# The COVID-19 Catastrophe

For those whose lives were lost to COVID-19

# The COVID-19 Catastrophe

What's Gone Wrong and How to Stop it Happening Again

## Richard Horton

polity

First published in 2020 by Polity Press

Polity Press
65 Bridge Street
Cambridge CB2 1UR, UK

Polity Press
101 Station Landing
Suite 300
Medford, MA 02155, USA

ISBN-13: 978-1-5095-4645-9
ISBN-13: 978-1-5095-4646-6 (pb)

A catalogue record for this book is available from the British Library.

Typeset in 12/15 Fournier MT by
Servis Filmsetting Ltd, Stockport, Cheshire

For further information on Polity, visit our website:
politybooks.com

# Contents

Fear can be considered the basis for all human civilization.

Lars Svendsen, *The Philosophy of Fear* (2008)

# Preface

COVID-19 is a pandemic of paradoxes.

Most of those who became infected with this new coronavirus suffered only mild disease, perhaps not easily shaken off, yet shaken off nevertheless. But a substantial number – perhaps as many as one in five – developed a much more severe illness, often requiring intensive care and mechanical ventilation. For far too many, COVID-19 meant that death was their destiny.

Being older and living with chronic disease were important risks for worse outcomes. Yet a significant proportion of those who endured severe illness were also young and previously fit and well.

The scientific community made an astonishing contribution to producing the new knowledge needed to guide a response to COVID-19. But many questions about the virus and the disease it causes remain unanswered, leaving important gaps in our understanding of the pandemic that make its control exceptionally difficult.

The World Health Organization (WHO) acted with unprecedented velocity to declare a Public Health Emergency of International Concern (PHEIC). But the world's only global health agency also struggled under intolerable political pressures to retain its credibility.

Countries pledged their support to international cooperation to defeat the pandemic. Yet those same countries were embarrassingly slow to match words with deeds, and too often they resorted to rivalry and blame.

This was a pandemic that was described and reported in terms of statistics – numbers of infections, numbers of patients in critical care and numbers of deaths. Lives were transformed into mathematical summaries. Graphs of the epidemic were drawn. And countries were compared for their rates of mortality.

But those who died must not be summarised. They must not become lines on squared paper. They must not become mere rates used to argue differences between nations. Every death counts. A person who died in Wuhan is as important as one who died in New York. Our way of describing the impact of the pandemic erased the biographies of the dead. The science and politics of COVID-19 became exercises in radical dehumanisation.

At press conference after press conference, government ministers and their medical and scientific advisors described the deaths of their neighbours as 'unfortunate'. But these were not unfortunate deaths. They were not unlucky, inappropriate or even regrettable. Every death was evidence of systematic government misconduct – reckless acts of omission that constituted breaches in the duties of public office.

I edit a medical journal, *The Lancet*, which found itself a conduit between medical scientists desperately trying to understand

COVID-19 and politicians and policymakers charged with responding to the pandemic. As we read and published the work of these remarkable frontline workers, I was struck by the gap between the accumulating evidence of scientists and the practice of governments. As this space grew larger, I became angry. Missed opportunities and appalling misjudgements were leading to the avoidable deaths of tens of thousands of citizens. There had to be a reckoning.

This book is their story.

# Acknowledgements

I wrote this short book under lockdown in London. I owe a debt of thanks to many people. To Ingrid Wolfe, who welcomed me home. To Isobel and Aleem. To Laura, live long. To my colleagues at *The Lancet* who worked tirelessly to ensure that the most reliable research on COVID-19 was peer reviewed and published rapidly to support those responding on the frontlines of this pandemic. To the scientists in China, Hong Kong, Italy, the UK and elsewhere who took time under immense pressure and difficulty to describe their extraordinary experiences. To John Thompson, who took a chance. To Emma Longstaff, Helen Davies, Lucas Jones, Neil de Cort and Caroline Richmond from Polity, who helped to make the message real. And to three anonymous reviewers, whose comments and suggestions helped to sharpen the substance of my argument. As we have all learned to say: stay safe, stay strong.

# I

# From Wuhan to the World

> While the human race battles itself, fighting over ever more crowded turf and scarcer resources, the advantage moves to the microbes' court. They are our predators and they will be victorious if we, Homo sapiens, do not learn how to live in a rational global village that affords the microbes few opportunities.
>
> It's either that or we brace ourselves for the coming plague.
>
> Laurie Garrett, *The Coming Plague* (1994)

Something happened. The precise details still remain uncertain and may never be fully uncovered. But here is what one can reasonably be sure of so far.

On 30 December 2019, samples were taken from the lungs of a patient with a mysterious pneumonia. He had been admitted to Wuhan Jin Yin-tan Hospital in Wuhan, Hubei Province, China. A test called real-time reverse transcriptase polymerase chain reaction (RT-PCR) confirmed the presence of a new type of coronavirus.

Coronaviruses are common in animals, such as bats, cats and camels. There are hundreds of different types of coronavirus. Six had been known to infect human beings – spillover infections into humans from their animal hosts. They are responsible for around 10 to 15 per cent of cases of the common cold.

Four human coronaviruses cause only mild to moderate symptoms – NL63 (identified in the Netherlands in 2004), HKU1 (discovered in Hong Kong in 2005) and OC43 and 229E (both major causes of the common cold). But two coronaviruses pose much more serious threats to human health – Severe Acute Respiratory Syndrome coronavirus (SARS-CoV-1) and Middle-East Respiratory Syndrome coronavirus (MERS-CoV). Could the virus discovered in Wuhan be a seventh and also more dangerous type of coronavirus?

The genetic code of the novel virus was quickly sequenced. Comparisons with existing viral genomes showed that it was closely related to a bat SARS-like strain. Those four letters – S-A-R-S – struck fear and not a little panic into Chinese health officials when the news arrived in Beijing. An outbreak of SARS in 2002–3 had infected 8,096 people and caused 774 deaths across 37 countries (a disturbingly high 10 per cent mortality rate). The political mishandling of that epidemic had brought widespread international criticism of China's leaders. A repeat of that national humiliation could not be allowed.

The early response to the discovery of this new SARS-like virus, eventually named SARS-CoV-2, was one of paralysing anxiety. Li Wenliang was working as an ophthalmologist in Wuhan. On 30 December, he privately alerted medical friends and colleagues through his WeChat account about the existence of the new SARS virus. When his online posts leaked and reached the local Wuhan police, he was detained, questioned and admonished for 'rumour-mongering'. Li was forced to sign a statement confirming that he would stop spreading these alleged rumours. Local Communist Party officials in China like to keep a low profile with Beijing. Post-Tiananmen, their primary duty is to preserve public order and stability. In their eyes, Li Wenliang had to be gagged.

Meanwhile, a health alert was released by Wuhan's local government authorities on 31 December. Doctors in Wuhan had noticed that several patients admitted to hospital with this new virus-like disease shared a common story – they had all visited Huanan seafood market, a live-animal and seafood wholesale market in the city. The source of the original SARS outbreak in 2002–3 was eventually traced to civets, cat-like mammals that resemble ferrets, which had in turn become infected from bats. Was the same sequence of events now repeating itself? Had the new SARS-like virus again jumped from animals to humans (this type of species transfer is called a zoonotic infection)? It seemed likely. The market was shut down on 1 January.

The Chinese government had learned lessons from 2002–3. As soon as Beijing officials received the report from Wuhan, they informed the World Health Organization's country office in the city. On 1 January, WHO set up an Incident Management Support Team to investigate the outbreak. By 3 January, 44 cases of the new disease had been reported. Worryingly, these patients were not suffering from the common cold. Eleven had very severe pneumonia.

The next day, WHO alerted the world to this outbreak

via Twitter: 'China has reported to WHO a cluster of pneumonia cases – with no deaths – in Wuhan, Hubei Province. Investigations are underway to identify the cause of this illness.' On 5 January, the agency made a more formal official notification of the outbreak, and on 10 January it issued technical guidance about how to detect, test and manage new cases of the disease.

Twenty years after the first outbreak of SARS, Chinese science was far better prepared. The country's scientists quickly isolated the virus and sequenced its genome, which they shared publicly on 12 January.

The next day, the first case of infection outside China was reported – WHO issued a statement saying that a traveller from Wuhan had arrived in Thailand and had been hospitalised on 8 January. It emphasised that 'The possibility of cases being identified in other countries was not unexpected, and reinforces why WHO calls for ongoing active monitoring and preparedness in other countries.'

Dr Tedros Adhanom Ghebreyesus, WHO's director-general, now realised he had the makings of a health crisis on his hands. His predecessor, Dr Margaret Chan, had been criticised for being slow to respond to the outbreak of Ebola virus in West Africa, which began in December 2013. That outbreak led to over 11,000 reported deaths. Like China over SARS, WHO could not afford to be seen to fail again. The agency said that Dr Tedros 'will consult with Emergency Committee members and could call for a meeting of the committee on short notice.'

The committee in question was the International Health Regulations (IHR) Emergency Committee. The IHR are legally binding rules designed 'to prevent, protect against, control, and provide a public health response to the international spread of disease.' If a disease endangers international public health, the committee can recommend, and the director-general of WHO can issue, a Public Health Emergency of International Concern (PHEIC).

The declaration of a PHEIC is, in the words of the IHR, 'an extraordinary event'. It is probably the most extraordinary power that a director-general of WHO possesses. Although they must consult a country about a disease threat, they are free to ignore their views or wishes. It is the decision of the director-general alone as to whether there is enough evidence for a PHEIC to be issued. This is serious power.

Ebola was first reported in Guinea in December 2013, before spreading to Liberia and Sierra Leone. The case fatality was 40 per cent. Individuals with Ebola virus disease were identified in Mali and Nigeria. The infection was also transported to the US, the UK, Italy and Spain. Dr Chan declared a PHEIC on 8 August 2014, eight months after the first cases of Ebola were described. The need to avoid a similar delay would have weighed heavily on the mind of Dr Tedros. He needed to evaluate the available evidence about what was happening in Wuhan carefully, but also quickly.

There are two criteria that must be met for a PHEIC to be declared. First, the disease must constitute a public health risk to other states through the international spread of that disease.

Second, the disease must potentially require a coordinated international response in order to control it.

At the first Emergency Committee meeting on 22–3 January 2020, members were evenly split as to whether they should recommend a PHEIC. Many informed observers were surprised. When the threat of a new infectious disease emerges, the common view, based on past failures, is that one should have a very low threshold for calling a global red alert. But Dr Tedros paused. Without the backing of the Emergency Committee he wasn't prepared to act alone. He needed more evidence – and time.

His anxieties only worsened when, on 24 January, a team of Hong Kong scientists published findings showing that the novel coronavirus could be transmitted from person to person. Ominously, they directly compared the new outbreak with the 2002–3 SARS epidemic, and they made several important recommendations:

> Learning from the SARS outbreak, which started as animal-to-human transmission during the first phase of the epidemic, all game meat trades should be optimally regulated to terminate this portal of transmission. But ... it is still crucial to isolate patients and trace and quarantine contacts as early as possible because symptomatic infection appears possible ..., educate the public on both food and personal hygiene, and alert health-care workers on compliance to infection control.[1]

While scientists were dissecting the genetics and biology of the virus, doctors were struggling to manage the disease it caused.

This condition was no straightforward pneumonia. Although many patients who contracted the infection had a mild illness and recovered quickly, a large subgroup (around 20 per cent) developed a much more severe form of the disease. Common presenting symptoms were fever, cough, muscle pain and fatigue. But if you were male, older and had a pre-existing disease, such as diabetes, high blood pressure, obesity or a heart condition, you seemed more likely to become critically ill – and die.

The onset of severe illness was usually heralded by shortness of breath about a week after the initial symptoms. There then ensued a rapid progression to acute respiratory distress syndrome, requiring mechanical ventilation on an intensive care unit (ICU). And then a pathological explosion took place. A storm of chemicals called cytokines were released by the body. Patients developed multiple organ failures – acute injuries of the heart, kidneys and liver, blood clots in small vessels, and secondary infections. All doctors could do was mechanically ventilate and support patients on ICU as best they could and hope they pulled through. Half of those admitted to ICU didn't.

The first clinical description of the disease, which would later be called COVID-19, was also published on 24 January.[2] The authors of that report were clearly alarmed by what they were seeing. They described a 'serious, sometimes fatal, pneumonia' that 'required ICU admission'. They reported that 'The number of deaths is rising quickly' and noted that 'Airborne precautions, such as a fit-tested N95 respirator, and other personal protective equipment are strongly recommended.' They underlined the fact that COVID-19 shared 'some resemblance to SARS-CoV and MERS-CoV infections.' They emphasised that no treatment existed. And they stressed 'the pandemic potential' of the new coronavirus.

Dr Tedros visited China and met President Xi Jinping on 28 January. He was beginning to understand the enormous gravity of the outbreak, and on 30 January he reconvened the IHR Emergency Committee. This time there was no split. The committee recommended action. Dr Tedros declared a PHEIC the same day. In WHO's own words, a PHEIC 'implies a situation that: is serious, unusual, or unexpected; carries implications for public health beyond the affected State's national border; and may require immediate international action.'

It had taken thirty days, not eight months, to issue WHO's highest category of international alert. The world had been warned. And it was still only January.

The 'pandemic potential' of SARS-CoV-2 was further highlighted by Gabriel Leung and a team of scientists at the University of Hong Kong on 31 January. They too understood the danger the world faced. As the capital city of Hubei Province, Wuhan is a major domestic and international transport hub. Flights out of Wuhan carried passengers to Bangkok, Hong Kong, Seoul, Singapore, Tokyo, Taipei, Kuala Lumpur, Sydney, Melbourne and London. It was no accident that the first reported case of infection outside of China was in Thailand.

Leung and his team calculated that human-to-human spread of SARS-CoV-2 was already taking place in multiple Chinese cities. Worse, though, they warned that, 'on the present trajectory, [SARS-CoV-2] could be about to become a global epidemic in the absence of mitigation.' They recommended that, 'To possibly succeed [in preventing a pandemic], substantial, even draconian measures that limit population mobility should be seriously and immediately considered in affected areas, as should strategies to drastically reduce within-population contact rates through cancellation of mass gatherings, school closures, and instituting working-from-home arrangements ...'

They urged the closing of live-animal markets and the acceleration of vaccine development. And they exhorted that 'preparedness plans should be readied for deployment at short notice, including securing supply chains of pharmaceuticals, personal protective equipment, hospital supplies, and the necessary human resources to deal with the consequences of a global outbreak of this magnitude.'[3] Governments had been cautioned.

\*

As Adam Kucharski argues in *The Rules of Contagion*, 'If you've seen one pandemic, you've seen ... one pandemic.'[4] His point is that every pandemic has unique characteristics, which mean that generalisations are very hard to make. But there are several crucial features of infections that do reliably influence their propensity to spread.

One critical measure of pandemic potential is the reproduction number, or $R_0$. This figure represents the expected number of infections produced by a primary case in a completely susceptible population. If the Ro is two, then one case becomes two, two becomes four, four becomes eight, and so on. If Ro<1, the epidemic will eventually die out.

The Wuhan outbreak of SARS-CoV-2 began with an Ro of around 2.4.[5] That is, it had a high potential for epidemic spread. And spread it did – by direct contact with people who had the infection, including breathing in droplets from the nose or mouth of a person who is infected, or by touching objects or surfaces on which the virus had landed. In a report from the Chinese Center for Disease Control and Prevention describing the early trajectory of the epidemic, Chinese scientists emphasised that 'this novel coronavirus is highly contagious.' They went on,

> It has spread extremely rapidly from a single city to the entire country within only about 30 days. Moreover, it has achieved such far-reaching effects even in the face of extreme response measures including the complete shutdown and isolation of whole cities, cancellation of Chinese New Year celebrations, prohibition of attendance at school and work, massive mobilisation of health and public health personnel as well as military medical units, and rapid construction of entire hospitals.[6]

On 23 January, Chinese authorities locked down Wuhan, cutting off all transportation links. Mass quarantine was extended to a total of 36 million people across thirteen additional cities shortly thereafter. But, by then, it was too late. After Thailand, cases transported from Wuhan were reported in Japan, South Korea, the US, Canada, Nepal, Hong Kong, Singapore, Malaysia and Taiwan. The virus tracked rail and air transportation routes out of Wuhan.

The first European cases arrived in France on 24 January, in Germany, on 27 January. The first cases in the UK were described on 31 January.The first death outside China took place in the Philippines on 2 February. On 3 February, the cruise ship *Diamond Princess* was quarantined off Yokohama, Japan. A viral fire had been ignited and it was spreading unchecked around the world.

Italy endured the first humanitarian catastrophe outside of China. The country went into a nationwide lockdown on 9 March. The entire Lombardy region (16 million people) was placed in quarantine. If you left home, you had to carry a certificate explaining the reason for your excursion. Those who violated the lockdown faced fines of between €400 and €3000.

Spain also suffered an unspeakably traumatic epidemic. The country went into lockdown on 14 March. France (full) and Germany (partial) implemented lockdowns shortly after – on 17 March and 22 March, respectively. The UK was slower than some of its European neighbours but eventually switched off its economy on 24 March. The British public already knew what was coming. They had begun to change their behaviour well before lockdown became official government policy. UK politicians were behind the public curve. On 27 March, Prime Minister Boris Johnson announced that he had contracted the infection.

The response in the US was predictably unpredictable. The first imported case was reported from Washington state on 21 January. President Trump initially called SARS-CoV-2 'the new hoax'. By 30 January, he was describing the epidemic as 'pretty much under control'. By 2 February, his administration had 'pretty much shut it down.' By 27 February, 'it will disappear.' On 4 March, he claimed there were 'very small numbers in the US'. 10 March: 'It's really working out.' 12 March: 'It's going to go away.' But, by 17 March, President Trump was forced to admit – 'This is a pandemic.'

Nowhere was spared. WHO reported that 213 countries, areas or territories were affected, from India to Indonesia, from Turkey to Algeria, and from Brazil to Ecuador. No country tested every member of its population, so it is impossible to be precise about the exact number of infections that took place worldwide. Deaths are a more reliable measure, since in many countries there are more formal means of death certification which can be assembled into national mortality statistics. But, even using deaths as a metric, one should be concerned and cautious about the accuracy of data – such as those from Russia, Iran and China.

China revised its numbers upwards by 50 per cent in April, adding a further 1,290 fatalities to the total reported for Wuhan. And even then it is likely that the total number of deaths reported for China is an underestimate. When account was taken of the changing case definitions China used as its epidemic evolved, one study put the total number of cases at 232,000.

At the time of writing (May 2020), the number of confirmed cases of SARS-CoV-2 stood at 5,204,508. That is more than the populations of Panama, Kuwait, Croatia, or ten countries in sub-Saharan Africa.

The total number of deaths stood at 337,687. The nations with most deaths, as reported by WHO, were:

| | |
|---|---|
| US | 94,011 |
| UK | 36,675 |
| Italy | 32,735 |
| Spain | 28,678 |
| France | 28,281 |
| Brazil | 21,048 |
| Belgium | 9,237 |
| Germany | 8,247 |
| Iran | 7,359 |
| Mexico | 6,989 |
| Canada | 6,277 |
| Netherlands | 5,811 |

The global distribution of infection is highly uneven. As of 25 May 2020, the Americas had recorded 2,338,124 cases of SARS-CoV-2. Europe was close behind, with 2,006,984 cases. Then came the Arab World (415,806 cases), South-East Asia (191,966 cases) and the Western Pacific (173,621 cases). Africa has not been spared either – 77,295 cases have been reported, although that number is certainly an underestimate. One report from WHO's regional office in Brazzaville estimated that as many as 190,000 Africans could eventually die from COVID-19.

The public health response to this highly contagious virus – called non-pharmaceutical interventions – was initially implemented reluctantly in most Western democracies, and even then in incremental steps. First came advice to wash hands regularly and properly (singing 'Happy Birthday' twice), improve cough etiquette, avoid touching your face, and use and then dispose of paper tissues. Next came a recommendation to practise physical distancing and reduce social mixing – at a minimum, avoid shaking hands, hugging, or kissing non-family members. Finally, lockdown – the almost complete closure of entire cultures.

School terms ended abruptly. Universities sent students home. Restaurants put up their shutters. Theatres cancelled productions. Museums locked their doors. Not even local libraries and churches were exempted. Weddings, baptisms and sporting events were all banned. The retail businesses allowed to remain open were pharmacies, food and hardware stores, supermarkets, petrol stations, bicycle shops, launderettes, garages, car rentals, pet shops, newsagents, post offices and banks. The only reasons you were allowed to leave home, unless you were a key worker (in health and social care, education and childcare, food and necessary goods, local and national government, utilities, public safety and national security, and transport), were to buy essential necessities (as infrequently as possible), visit a doctor or vulnerable person, donate blood, and exercise once a day.

But although the decision to go into full lockdown was hard, it was even harder to decide how to return society to some semblance of normal functioning. In the UK, just three weeks into its lockdown, public debate was already focusing on an exit strategy. But, without either a vaccine to confer immunity or adequate capacity to test, trace and isolate contacts, the prospects for an early exit were nothing more than speculation mixed with touches of fantasy and delusion.

The evidence from Wuhan was sobering.[7] Around 90 per cent of the workforce had been locked down. Assuming an Ro of over 2 and with a phased return to work (25 per cent of the workforce returning during the two weeks after lockdown ends, then 50 per cent during the next two weeks, and finally 100 per cent returning to work), epidemiologists from the London School of Hygiene and Tropical Medicine calculated that it would be safe to start lifting intense physical distancing measures only in early April. If lockdown was lifted either prematurely or completely, the risk of a second wave of infection flaring up was almost guaranteed.

Since Wuhan's lockdown began on 23 January, that meant at least ten weeks of the most extreme measures to extinguish virus transmission. Wuhan did cautiously start lifting its restrictions on social mixing on 8 April. But many schools, shops and cinemas remained closed.

Gabriel Leung, who correctly predicted that a global pandemic would ensue from the events in Wuhan, was working intensively to define what an exit strategy should look like.[8] He and his team in Hong Kong warned against relaxing restrictions too soon. If the Ro crept above 1 again, a second wave of the pandemic would be inevitable. He advised resuming economic activity in lockdown settings under what he called an Ro<1 constraint. He also advised continuous surveillance of two critical measures – the Case Fatality Risk and Rt (the instantaneous reproduction number, or the R value at a particular time and place).

The Case Fatality Risk is the ratio of laboratory-confirmed deaths to confirmed cases. It will vary according to the preexisting levels of health of a population and the availability of healthcare resources. It could be a valuable measure of the health system's ability to treat severe cases of the infection.

Rt would be a sensitive indicator to tell whether the epidemic is resurfacing. Real-time monitoring of Rt will depend on implementing community testing for the early detection of infection, with subsequent contact tracing if someone is found to have the virus, and then quarantine to prevent possible further transmission. Digital monitoring of levels of social mixing could also be helpful.

But maybe the truth is that life will never fully return to normal until a vaccine becomes available – and perhaps not even then. A vaccine is not a 'magic bullet'. It is unlikely to be completely effective, and it is unlikely to be taken up by every citizen. Perhaps COVID-19 represents an impermeable boundary between one moment in our lives and another. We can never go back.

\*

If human life has been so affected, so acutely and so suddenly by this coronavirus, it seems important to ask what the political, economic, social and cultural consequences might be. It is too soon to be sure, of course. But, even while the pandemic was raging through countries, some fiery judgements were being made nevertheless.

David Nabarro, WHO's special envoy for COVID-19, announced with considerable drama on 13 April, 'This virus isn't going to go away … Yes, we will have to wear masks. There will be more physical distancing … It's a revolution.'

Lockdown has certainly changed the way we interact with one another. Walking down the street we may cross the road if we see someone else walking towards us. We want to maintain our 2-metre separation. We queue on the road to get into the supermarket, sometimes waiting over an hour before being allowed to enter. Numbers of shoppers are strictly limited in each store. And we are now used to seeing our fellow citizens wearing masks and rubber gloves. They may back away from us if we come too close or dive into another shopping aisle if we inadvertently turn into their path. Everyone is potentially infected and so everyone is a risk. We can only rely on the safety of our immediate household.

Are these new behaviours simply examples of wise caution at a time of danger? Or do they represent a catastrophic loss of social trust, a fissuring in our communities, a fragmentation of our solidarity? Is that the revolution we have to look forward to?

One revolution certainly did take place – in our working

lives. For some of us, the fortunate ones, those who didn't have to earn our living on the frontline of risk, home – the kitchen table, the sofa or even the bed – became our new office. While working from home might have attractions, the degree of isolation we live with has important implications for mental health.

Samantha Brooks and her colleagues at the Department of Psychological Medicine, King's College London, have reviewed the world literature on the impacts of quarantine. Their findings are alarming.[9] Isolation can cause post-traumatic stress, confusion, fear, anger, frustration and, of course, boredom. Some of these effects will be long-lasting. They recommended that periods of isolation should be as short as possible. Working from home might be a welcome pleasure at first. But it also carries the seeds of sometimes severe mental trauma.

Democracy also shifted. Parliaments were suspended. Politicians often deployed war-like language ('We are at war with an invisible killer'), with invocations to 'pull together', conjure up our 'Dunkirk sprit' and 'fight' the virus.

War metaphors carry huge emotional force. They are widely understood by the public. Words of war convey a sense of threat, urgency and risk. They suggest a battle with an evil enemy. The stakes are high. Sacrifices will have to be made. But war metaphors have their own dangers. They can create an atmosphere where dissent and criticism of government policy are discouraged, possibly even branded as a kind of betrayal. They emphasise treatment, not prevention. Turning the strategy to tackle a disease into a battlefield could worsen the mental health of those caught in the middle of the 'war zone'. And the idea of war also implies victory or defeat – where neither may be the likely outcome with a virus that is here to stay.

China became a particular focus for comment. Some heaped praise on China's response to SARS-CoV-2. 'We appreciate the seriousness with which China is taking this outbreak,' said Dr Tedros on 28 January. Controversially, he has continued to thank the Chinese government for taking 'action massively at the epicentre, at the source of the outbreak … and that helped in preventing cases from being exported to other provinces in China and the rest of the world.'

But others have been less happy with China's tactics. Tom Tugendhat is a British Conservative MP who chairs the influential Parliamentary Foreign Affairs Select Committee. He was scathing about China's coronavirus response. On 13 April, as Wuhan opened up and as the UK was passing through the peak of its deaths, he commented that 'China has deliberately lied in order to preserve the strength of the [Communist] Party at the expense of its people.'

The verdict on the virtues of China's response remains to be written. There are legitimate questions the Chinese government must answer. There is a gap in the timeline of the pandemic outbreak. The earliest known cases reported in China were first described in early December 2019. Beijing informed WHO on 31 December. What happened during the intervening period? What really took place in Wuhan in December? Did local Communist Party officials suppress evidence of a new virus? Did they delay telling the national government in Beijing?

Also, why did Chinese authorities tell WHO on 11–12 January that no additional cases of COVID-19 had been detected since 3 January? That statement was plainly untrue. Was Beijing complicit in playing down the significance of the outbreak? The Chinese government refutes all criticism.

On 2 February, I received an email entitled 'A desperate plea from an ordinary citizen in China'. The writer called herself Moona. This is what she wrote about living in China during the time of coronavirus:

> Currently, there are at least five cities, including Wuhan, that have suspended the public transport system; ten provinces and cities, including Hubei and Beijing, that have shut down road passenger transport; 16 provinces that have suspended inter-provincial passenger transport; and many cities in 28 provinces that have completely or partially suspended urban public transportation. Yesterday, Huanggang issued a notice ordering a house quarantine for all urban households, allowing only a designated family member to shop for essentials once in every two days. The news and constant updates include messages from my local government telling me that many cities have made it mandatory to wear a mask in public or for using public transport. But masks have sold out so quickly in many smaller cities (and online as well), while prices have gone up twenty times. In short, if you are poor, you're more than likely to not get a mask at all – and it's usually the poor who cannot afford to stop working.
>
> At 7:30 pm yesterday, Hangzhou became the first city in China to issue a free mask policy for its citizens in seven urban districts to

alleviate the problem that has been the elephant in the room, with an online reservation system for five masks for each person every ten days. Even Wuhan hasn't implemented any government policy like this to help its citizens. So access to masks largely depends on donations and self-help by local communities. The bottom line is, a large population in China is suffering, not just from the virus but from the resulting isolation, high uncertainty, anxiety and stress, reduced resources and freedom for daily living, and loss of income. And the point on income really should be considered. With weak social protection in China, in conjunction with the estimate of 60% of labour engaged in the informal economy in Asian and Pacific developing countries, lack of employment benefits and protection renders people extremely vulnerable to crises, such as the current one. There would have been social outcries if this happened in any other Western country, but just because there isn't an outcry in China doesn't make its people lesser people who shouldn't be treated any less. If anything, it shows how deeply the population has been culturally and politically suppressed, and how the voice of the really poor in China gets completely buried and forgotten. This just isn't right.

In a crisis like this, it hurts me so much to see that it's (once again) the well-off who get priority and consideration. Those who actually do not have the ability or resources to take care of themselves inevitably get left behind. Government policies are understandably a combination of politics, economics, sociology, and international relations. But equality to health gets thrown out of the picture in the middle of all these, even in scholarship. This cannot be right. The top health journals should be redirected toward a more compassionate and sensitive discourse. *The Lancet* please do something, somebody please do something. In a practical sense, the government cares about its 'face' more than anything; if there was a prominent international voice calling for it to look into something it just might ... and that's all that the suppressed and the poor have for hope. So please, help. I understand this might be an effort in vain, but I really hope it is not. So here it is, a desperate plea, and I really hope this message sees you in good time.

The Chinese government owes the world a more detailed explanation of what took place in Wuhan. I don't care what we call it – an international inquiry, a fact-finding mission, truth and reconciliation. I don't seek blame. I don't want punishment. I simply want to know what happened. Something happened. We need to know so that we have the best chance of preventing it from happening again.

But I also believe that we must say this – Chinese scientists and health workers deserve our gratitude. I know from my own knowledge of these dedicated individuals that they worked tirelessly to understand the nature of this pandemic. They made it their duty to inform WHO when they were sure there was reason to signal global alarm. And, in my dealings with Chinese scientists and policymakers, I have observed nothing less than an extraordinary commitment to collaborate openly and unconditionally to defeat this disease.

\*

Despite the uncertainties – and there are many, since we are still in the early phase of understanding this disease – perhaps we do know enough to draw two conclusions.

First, much attention was given to the celebrities who contracted SARS-CoV-2 – Marianne Faithful, Tom Hanks and Rita Wilson, Idris Elba, Sophie Trudeau, Prince Albert of Monaco and Prince Charles in the UK. It was easy to think the virus was a threat to everyone equally. But that was not the case. COVID-19 overwhelmingly affected those who were poorer, less able and sicker. There was a steep social gradient to this disease. And it seemed to affect black and minority ethnic communities especially badly. Those on the frontlines of care were particularly vulnerable and often unprotected. COVID-19 exploited and worsened already existing inequalities in society.

Second, before COVID-19, the idea of a 'key worker' was probably a rather obscure notion in the public's mind. No longer. Just as 'first responders' after 9/11 – firefighters, police officers and emergency medical workers – became heroic symbols of a country under terrorist attack, so key workers came to embody the commitment of those without whom society really would have collapsed.

The essential services key workers provide – whether they were health workers dispensing care, people working in supermarkets ensuring continuous supplies of food, or those delivering vital services, from refuse collection to public utilities – became the resilient and moral backbone of the response worldwide. It was these key workers who kept countries going while the rest of us languished at home. It was these key workers who saved the lives of the sick and protected the lives of the poor and vulnerable. It was these key workers, so often overlooked and taken for granted, who, as we now realised, are the real foundation for public order and public safety. We truly do owe them our lives.

## 2

# Why Were We Not Prepared?

We need to accept that the timing of a disaster's occurrence is unambiguously random.

Lucy Jones, *The Big Ones* (2018)

'We were poorly prepared.' Ian Boyd was writing in *Nature* in March 2020.[1] He had been one of the UK's government's chief scientific advisers from 2012 to 2019 and recalled taking part in a 'practice run' for an influenza pandemic. 200,000 people died in this simulation. 'It left me shattered.' Did government learn from this experiment to identify critical weaknesses in the national response to an epidemic? Boyd notes, ruefully, 'We learnt what would help, but did not necessarily implement those lessons.'

Boyd was alluding to Exercise Cygnus – scenario planning for a pandemic influenza outbreak that took place in October 2016. Pandemic influenza is top of the UK government's National Risk Register. A pandemic is deemed the most severe civil emergency risk to our society. The same is true for most Western democracies. The result of Cygnus was a stark warning: UK preparedness was 'currently not sufficient to cope with the extreme demands of a severe epidemic.'

National failings were sometimes sublimated into international attacks. In a remarkable speech given at the White House on 14 April, President Donald Trump issued an instruction 'to halt funding of the World Health Organization while a review is conducted to assess the World Health Organization's role in severely mismanaging and covering up the spread of the coronavirus.' This was an astonishing allegation. An American president was charging WHO with nothing less than murder – 'so much death has been caused by their mistakes.' His case against WHO was incendiary and is worth quoting at length. The speech will become a key historical document in the history of this pandemic.

One of the most dangerous and costly decisions from the WHO was its disastrous decision to oppose travel restrictions from China and other nations ... The WHO's attack on travel restrictions put political correctness above life-saving measures ... The reality is that the WHO failed to adequately obtain, vet, and share information in a timely and transparent fashion ... The WHO failed in this basic duty and must be held accountable ... The WHO failed to investigate credible reports from sources in Wuhan that conflicted directly with the Chinese government's official accounts. There was credible information to suspect human-to-human transmission in December, 2019, which should have spurred the WHO to investigate and investigate immediately. Through the middle of January it parroted and publicly endorsed the idea that there was not human-to-human transmission happening, despite reports and clear evidence to the contrary. The delays that WHO experienced in declaring a public health emergency cost valuable time ... The inability of the WHO to obtain virus samples to this date has deprived the scientific community of essential data ... Had the WHO done its job to get medical experts into China to objectively assess the situation on the ground and to call out China's lack of transparency the outbreak could have been contained at its source with very little death, very little death, and certainly very little death by comparison. This would have saved thousands of lives and avoided worldwide economic damage. Instead, the WHO willingly took China's assurances at face value and ... defended the actions of the Chinese government, even praising China for its so-called transparency – I don't think so. The WHO pushed China's misinformation about the virus, saying it was not communicable and there was no need for travel bans ... The WHO's reliance on China's disclosures likely caused a twenty-fold increase in cases worldwide and it may be much more than that. The WHO has not addressed a single one of these concerns nor provided a serious explanation that acknowledges its own mistakes of which there were many.

I believe that President Trump's decision to cut funding to WHO in the middle of a global pandemic constituted a crime against humanity. Is that claim an exaggeration? No, and here is why. WHO exists to protect the health and wellbeing of the world's peoples. A crime against humanity is a knowing and inhumane attack against a people. By attacking and weakening WHO while the agency was doing all it could to protect peoples in some of the most vulnerable countries in the world, President

Trump has, in my view, met the criteria for the act of violence the international community calls a crime against humanity.

*

So who was responsible for a pandemic that infected over 5 million people and killed over 300,000? China? National governments? WHO? Some of the answers, I think, lie in the lessons from the last outbreak of a SARS virus in 2002–3.

In late 2002 in the southern Chinese province of Guangdong, a new coronavirus jumped from its animal host into humans. That event most likely took place in a live-animal market where a multiplicity of animals were caged, slaughtered, dismembered, and sold raw and cooked. These markets are crowded, busy and atrociously unhygienic. The likelihood of a virus making the transition from animal to human is high. The first known person to acquire the virus and to develop the associated disease it caused in November 2002 – an unusual type of pneumonia, the 'index case' – was from the city of Foshan.

Further outbreaks were reported in December. A Chinese team of scientists concluded in January 2003 that a new virus was probably responsible. They urged careful surveillance and reporting. But because their recommendations coincided with Chinese New Year they were either ignored or neglected. Not only was China's guard down, but the enormous numbers of people travelling home for New Year celebrations provided the perfect opportunity for the virus to spread. Which it did.

On 31 January in Guangzhou, a patient, ill and infected with this new virus, was admitted to one and then transferred to two further hospitals, passing the infection to around 200 people. As the number of those infected grew, news reached WHO. The agency's officials asked the Chinese government for details. They were told there was an outbreak of an acute respiratory illness that had affected 305 people, with five deaths.

Hong Kong suffered an outbreak of the new disease too. Twelve people staying at the Metropole Hotel fell sick with SARS in February 2003. They had contracted the virus from an infected doctor visiting from the Chinese mainland. Those twelve individuals returned home with the virus – to Singapore, Vietnam, Canada, Ireland and the US. Most of the more than 8,000 cases worldwide originated from this super-spreading moment. In March 2003, more than 300 people fell ill in the Amoy Gardens apartment towers.

By 12 March, under the leadership of the former Norwegian prime minister Gro Harlem Brundtland, WHO had issued a global alert. The responses from the affected countries were fast and impressive. Strict containment led to the extinguishing of the outbreak by May 2003. This particular coronavirus hasn't re-emerged since.

The outbreak was short, sharp and, although global, strictly confined to a very limited number of countries. But its effects had huge consequences. First, there was an enormous economic shock. Estimates put the short-term cost at US$80 billion, with China and Hong Kong especially badly hit. Second, there were implications for global health security. Health was no longer a minor or marginal political issue. Strengthening health systems now became a matter of national defence.

A further lesson was that epidemics such as SARS had to be fought internationally, as well as locally. The response to a virus that can spread so fast and furiously cannot be haphazard. It has to be coordinated. But the most cataclysmic lesson was political.

China performed poorly. The country's weak public health and primary healthcare systems, its turgid and authoritarian bureaucracy, excessive respect for political hierarchy, poor coordination, suppression of evidence, repression of the media, reluctance to ask for external assistance, and fear of internal instability all contributed to a less than optimal response. Chinese officials simply refused to share information with WHO. They practised a systematic deception.

On 16 April, WHO expressed 'strong concern over inadequate reporting' of SARS cases. It is rare for WHO to criticise one of its member states. But Brundtland's frustration was growing and, as a former prime minister, she had the confidence to call out the Chinese government. By 20 April 2003, China's minister of health and Beijing's mayor had both been fired by the new Chinese president, Hu Jintao. The government declared a 'nationwide war on SARS'. They vowed never to be shamed in the same way again.

The global response to SARS was judged a glorious success. By July, WHO was able to declare that the virus had been vanquished. As the respected US Institute of Medicine (IOM) concluded in 2004, 'the quality, speed, and effectiveness of the public health response to SARS brilliantly outshone past responses to international outbreaks of infectious disease, validating a decade's worth of progress in global public health networking.'[2]

This sense of achievement was matched with a warning. The IOM noted that SARS 'highlights the continuing need for investments in a robust response system that is prepared for the next emerging disease – whether naturally occurring or intentionally introduced.' Brundtland concluded that 'This is not the time to relax our vigilance. The world must remain on high alert for cases of SARS.'

The risk of a virally induced global humanitarian emergency was identified as a clear and present danger after SARS. The future required countries to build defences against a re-emergence of the virus – indeed, to prepare the world for the next pandemic of whatever kind. The most important demand was vigilance – a heightened and permanent state of awareness.

Practically, there must be a scientific readiness to identify the agent causing an outbreak, develop diagnostic tests, and discover new medicines and vaccines that could treat and eventually prevent the disease. The public health response that was needed was also clear – surveillance, early detection, isolation, contact tracing, quarantine, accumulating surge capacity within the health system to cope with what might be tens of thousands of severe infections, and effective communication to the public.

Modern quarantine means reducing the frequency of social contact, voluntary home curfew, cancelling mass gatherings, avoiding public transport, and closing public buildings and workplaces. These measures would introduce severe and unusual restrictions on the lives of most citizens. To win public acceptance, it would be essential to establish trust through rapid, regular and transparent communication, protect living standards through the provision of job security and compensation schemes, and maintain the morale of key workers. Finally, it was necessary to understand that SARS was 'a watershed event in the history of public health because of the degree of multinational cooperation to contain the disease'.[3]

Indeed, SARS represented the beginning of an entirely new geopolitical era. As noted by David Fidler, a specialist in international relations and global health law, 'SARS represents the first infectious disease to emerge into a radically new and different global political environment for public health.'[4] The 'historic moment' that was SARS came about because the coronavirus was 'the first post-Westphalian pathogen'.

The Peace of Westphalia in 1648 not only ended the Thirty Years' War but also initiated the birth of the modern nation-state. From 1648 until 2002–3, infectious diseases – indeed, all disease – could be managed largely within the confines of national borders. For over three centuries international relations were shaped by three principles: national sovereignty, non-intervention in the affairs of sovereign states, and consent-based international law.

Fidler described Westphalian governance as horizontal. It involved only states, focusing mainly on the details of how states should interact with one another. It made no attempt to address the way governments treated their own peoples. Countries might work together to strengthen their own national plans for tackling disease – for example, through the technical committees and resolutions passed at annual meetings of WHO – but SARS was the first occasion when sovereign states had to bend to the influence of non-state actors and global organisations, such as WHO.

Just as science, from Copernicus through Darwin to Einstein, has been an exercise in the gradual erosion of human vanity – the decentring of the human being from our understanding of the world – so pandemics have eroded governmental omnipotence. Nation-states have slowly had to succumb to curbs on their power and authority.

SARS was a different kind of pathogen because, like HIV, it posed a truly global threat. It became a global public health emergency. SARS inaugurated a new era of post-Westphalian public health – public health that transcended national borders and national sovereignties. And that new era itself was inaugurated with an achievement of spectacular proportions: 'the global campaign against SARS achieved a victory that will go down in the annals of public health and international relations history.'

Since SARS, there have been two further major outbreaks of zoonotic disease. One was Ebola in 2013. Countries and global agencies displayed disgraceful complacency in their lacklustre response to Ebola. A year earlier, another coronavirus – causing the Middle-East Respiratory Syndrome – hit Saudi Arabia and spread to Qatar and several other countries in the Arab world. Thankfully, the risk of person-to-person transmission was low and so MERS did not become the global threat that both SARS and Ebola posed. The world was not tested by MERS.

Zika was a different story. Transmitted by the bite of an infected *Aedes* mosquito and beginning in early 2015, Zika virus is suspected to have infected over half a million people, with most cases being reported in Brazil, Colombia, Venezuela, Martinique and Honduras. In February 2016, WHO declared a PHEIC in response to Zika virus. The epidemic ended in November 2016. But the tragedy of Zika is that the virus can be passed from a pregnant woman to her foetus, thereby causing an array of birth defects, notably microcephaly.

By the end of the West African Ebola and the Zika outbreaks in 2016, there was ample evidence to signal the urgent need for countries to strengthen their preparedness for new infectious pandemics. But, as WHO has described, fewer than half the countries of the world have the public health capacity to prevent or respond to new outbreaks of disease.[5] Any weak link in the global chain of preparedness and protection is a threat to all countries.

WHO warned, 'Many countries are struggling to sustain or develop their national preparedness capacities, primarily because of a lack of resources, competing national priorities, and a high turnover of health-care workers … Urgent action is needed to ensure that capacities are in place to prevent and manage health emergencies.' But these weaknesses were not addressed or prioritised by most nations. Even countries that were relatively well resourced – countries such as Italy, for example – found themselves engulfed by the consequences of

SARS-CoV-2. Partly, this failure to react to the threat can be explained by an understandable fear of the economic consequences of lockdowns. 'Milan does not stop,' said the mayor of Milan, Beppe Sala.

But the most important reason for the widespread complacency across much of Europe and North America was that political leaders underestimated the danger. They could not believe that a virus that originated in a Chinese city they had probably never heard of could have such calamitous effects in their own communities. Despite all of the evidence pointing to the devastating damage of recent infectious epidemics, this risk was just not on their horizon of possibilities.

The fact that this was so points to a miserable failure of government. Some political leaders have accepted and admitted these failures. As President Macron said on 13 April 2020, 'Were we ready? Obviously, not enough.'

In many countries, this lack of political vigilance was compounded by a decade of austerity economics that followed the global financial crisis of 2007–8. The Great Recession that ensued was one of the most severe downturns in the global economy since the Great Depression of the 1930s. Policies of austerity led to squeezed government budgets. And the health sector was often a particular victim of cuts in social spending.

In the UK after 2010, the National Health Service (NHS) saw an unprecedented decline in its growth at the same time as patient demand was increasing. Britain's public health system has endured £1 billion of cuts since 2015. Worse, the local infrastructure of public health, so essential for protecting communities from infection, was dismantled.

This reduction in growth in health spending was felt across most of Europe. Health services became steadily understaffed, short of resources, and stretched to breaking point, especially during winter months when patient demand was at its highest. In the decade leading up to COVID-19, the capacity of health systems could not keep pace with growing populations, ageing societies, changing patterns of disease and more expensive new treatments.

Despite President Trump's attempt to blame WHO and China for the destructive effects of COVID-19 on American society, it was the lack of readiness of the US public healthcare system that played a more important part. Public health departments nationally, in states and locally have been chronically underfunded. The Trump administration specifically targeted the US Centers for Disease Control and Prevention. Its budget was savaged, reducing epidemic prevention efforts across the world, including in China. The position of White House director for global health security and biothreats was axed by John Bolton, then national security advisor, in 2019, leaving no one to identify and call out the dangers of a global pandemic. The US was spectacularly unprepared for SARS-CoV-2, largely owing to its own acts of self-harm.

These turns away from investment in national and global health security reflect a larger trend: a general political antipathy to globalism – that is, an appreciation of the importance of international interdependence, solidarity and cooperation between nations and peoples. A decade of austerity created the conditions for politicians and their electorates to look inwards. Attending to the predicaments of one's own country is no bad thing. But there was a larger ideology at work.

Donald Trump in America, Brexit in the UK, Jair Bolsonaro in Brazil, Narendra Modi in India, Italy's Five Star Movement – each of these political watersheds stood for a departure from what had been, until the global financial crisis, a steady political alignment around a common global story: the need for greater international collaboration to solve some of the world's most pressing problems.

In the words of President Trump, speaking at the United Nations General Assembly in 2018, 'We reject the ideology of globalism, and we embrace the doctrine of patriotism.' And again, in 2019, 'The future does not belong to globalists, the future belongs to patriots.' But this narrow definition of patriotism ignored one brutal truth: viruses have no nationality.

The result of this turn away from globalism is that when SARS-CoV-2 arrived there was no global leadership, no willingness to cooperate, and no ability to view what was taking place as a lethal global challenge demanding a coordinated global response. Instead, there was inattention, rivalry and accusation.

\*

This brittle and dysfunctional 'international community' was also unprepared for a second epidemic – what has come to be called by WHO an 'infodemic'. An infodemic is an overflow of information, some of it true some of it not, which hampers a reliable and effective response to an epidemic. When confronted by a plethora of claims and counter-claims, who should one believe?

There have been debilitating examples of misinformation throughout the SARS-CoV-2 outbreak. These fall into four categories – first, conflicting theories about the cause of the disease. The view that this virus emerged as a zoonotic infection from a live-animal market in Wuhan has been challenged by several theories. The most conspiratorial is the claim that the virus was somehow engineered and then leaked from a biological weapons facility in the city. President Trump gave credence to the idea in April when he said, 'More and more we're hearing the story … We'll see.' Distracting attention away from the dangers of live-animal markets will only diminish the pressure to close those markets down. Another theory was that 5G wireless technology damaged human immune systems, thereby contributing to severe COVID-19 illness. 5G masts have been attacked and burnt down as a result. WHO has ruled that 5G signals pose no risk to human health, but still the idea persists.

A second source of misinformation concerns the symptoms of the illness and how the virus is transmitted. In India, some Hindu nationalists have sought to argue, incorrectly, that the Muslim community had tried to spread the virus deliberately to the Hindu population. They coined the terms 'corona-terrorism' and 'corona-Jihad', inciting discrimination, harassment and violence against Indian Muslims. Chinese citizens have also experienced overt racism and xenophobia, not helped by President Trump calling SARS-CoV-2 the 'Wuhan virus' and 'the plague from China'.

The third category of misinformation relates to alleged COVID-19 cures. There are by now hundreds of false stories of tests and treatments for this disease, including vitamin C, cocaine, marijuana and colloidal silver. And, finally, questions have been raised about what health authorities are doing to tackle the pandemic. One theory, widely circulated, has been that COVID-19 is largely an invention by the media and that the disease is no worse than a routine influenza epidemic – emphatically untrue.

WHO became so worried about the effects of an infodemic that it established a new unit – the Information Network for Epidemics, or EPI-WIN – to counter its impact.

But what is more sinister still is the part disinformation might have played in propagating false beliefs about COVID-19. Disinformation is that category of misinformation deliberately aimed to deceive. Those who propagate disinformation seek to amplify discord within societies. The European External Action Service has documented multiple examples of disinformation targeted at Europe and the European Union (EU). The intention behind these attacks is often to discredit the EU for the way it has handled the crisis, to suggest that the EU has failed to help its member states, and to show that other countries, such as China, have done more to help Europe than Europe itself. The false theories being distributed are typical, so the European External Action Service argues, of pro-Kremlin propaganda that aims 'to amplify divisions, sow distrust and chaos, and exacerbate crisis situations and issues of public concern.'

The answer as to why the world was unprepared for SARS-CoV-2 and COVID-19 has several further and even more disturbing twists, which I will discuss in the next three chapters. Collectively, these deficiencies in decision-making reflect not only the surprising fragility of modern science-based societies but also something far worse – inherent failures in the mechanics of Western democracies that threaten their very existence.

3

# Science: The Paradox of Success and Failure

A catalogue of the number of deaths induced by the major epidemics of historical times is staggering, and dwarfs the total deaths on all past battlefields.

Roy M. Anderson and Robert M. May, *Infectious Diseases of Humans* (1991)

The global scientific community made an unrivalled contribution to establishing a reliable foundation of knowledge to guide the response to the SARS-CoV-2 pandemic. And yet the management of COVID-19 represented, in many countries, the greatest science policy failure for a generation. What went wrong?

Before answering this question, one should acknowledge and applaud the successes. After enduring the global opprobrium following its handling of SARS, Chinese leaders invested heavily in their universities, and specifically in their capacities for scientific, technical and medical research. Confronted by a new virus, Chinese scientists were ready, equipped and swung quickly into action.

They reported the first 41 cases of COVID-19 in *The Lancet* on 24 January. The Chinese team was led by Bin Cao, a professor in the Department of Pulmonary and Critical Care Medicine at the China–Japan Friendship Hospital in Beijing. He assembled groups in Wuhan and Beijing which began to put together the epidemiological, clinical, laboratory and radiological data from this initial group of patients.[1]

Bin Cao and his colleagues provided the first case descriptions of symptoms and signs for COVID-19, an essential and urgent resource for doctors around the world facing patients with an unfamiliar type of pneumonia. They made the connection between the illness and exposure to the live-animal market. They described how a third of patients had to be admitted to intensive care. They calculated the average time from the onset of symptoms to ICU admission (10.5 days). They showed that patients often had blood profiles that revealed serious cardiac, renal and liver injuries. Chest computed tomography produced images that were abnormal in every case. One pattern of investigation was particularly disturbing – elevated levels of cytokines that constituted a 'cytokine storm'. The Chinese team described how some patients needed invasive mechanical ventilation and a special means to oxygenate blood when the lungs failed – a technique called extracorporeal membrane oxygenation. They also described how 15 per cent of the patients admitted to hospital had died.

The contrast between this impressive response and China's pitiful efforts during SARS in 2002–3 illustrates the remarkable scientific renaissance that had taken place in the country in just two decades. Bin Cao's team was not only able to gather state-of-the-art data on these early patients but also encouraged to write up their work, publish it free from censorship in foreign English-language medical journals, and make their findings available to others – all within weeks of the first reports of the new disease. The cultural, as well as the scientific, shift that had taken place in China was monumental.

Several further milestones were achieved by local scientific teams. Hong Kong clinicians working with colleagues in Shenzhen were the first to establish person-to-person transmission of SARS-CoV-2.[2] The genome sequence of the new virus was published on 29 January by a large team that included China's Center for Disease Control and Prevention, led by its president George Gao.[3] As I have already discussed, Gabriel Leung's group at the WHO Collaborating Centre for Infectious Disease Epidemiology and Control at the University of Hong Kong carefully documented the likelihood of a global epidemic.[4]

There were several urgent clinical questions that needed to be answered. Again, Chinese clinicians and scientists moved fast. Given the history of Zika virus and its effects on the foetus, one immediate question was whether this coronavirus could be transmitted from mother to baby. Joint teams from Wuhan and Beijing collaborated to study nine pregnant women who had COVID-19. Evidence of intrauterine vertical transmission was assessed by looking for SARS-CoV-2 in amniotic fluid, umbilical cord blood, breast milk and throat swabs from the newly born babies.[5] All women underwent Caesarean section and all survived. All nine children were born alive and well. None became infected with the virus. None of the samples taken for testing proved positive. Huijun Chen and his colleagues tentatively drew a preliminary but reassuring conclusion – there was no evidence that the virus could pass from mother to baby.

A further concern was the seriousness of COVID-19. The report of the first 41 patients indicated that one-third required admission to ICU and one in eight died. A report of 99 patients, published on 29 January, described an 11 per cent mortality rate among those admitted to hospital.[6] But more detailed descriptions of the severity of the illness were needed. How much should other countries be worried by this disease?

The early reports indicated that national health systems should be scaling up intensive care facilities, building stocks of personal protective equipment, and preparing for potentially high mortality. Wuhan's Jin Yin-tan hospital had been designated a specialist centre to treat patients with COVID-19. A team of doctors led by Professor You Shang reviewed their records and found that, out of 201 patients with confirmed COVID-19, 55 (27 per cent) became so critically ill that they required admission to ICU.[7] As they wrote on 21 February, 'During the outbreak of SARS-CoV-2 infection, the number of critically ill patients exceeded the capacity of ICUs. Therefore, two provisional ICUs were urgently established in Jin Yin-tan hospital.' But what they recorded was shocking – 62 per cent of the patients admitted to ICU died. Those who died were older (their average age was 65 years) and they developed multiple-organ failure. You Shang concluded that 'The mortality of critically ill patients with SARS-CoV-2 is considerable … The severity of SARS-CoV-2 pneumonia poses great strain on critical care resources in hospitals, especially if they are not adequately staffed or resourced.'

Between 16 and 24 February, a team from WHO visited China to assess the Chinese response to this coronavirus and to offer recommendations for countries not yet affected.[8] They concluded:

> In the face of a previously unknown virus, China has rolled out perhaps the most ambitious, agile and aggressive disease containment effort in history ... Achieving China's exceptional coverage with and adherence to these containment measures has only been possible due to the deep commitment of the Chinese people to collective action in the face of this common threat ... China's bold approach to contain the rapid spread of this new respiratory pathogen has changed the course of a rapidly escalating and deadly epidemic.

Central to this success was the 'series of major emergency research programs on virus genomics, antivirals, traditional Chinese medicines, clinical trials, vaccines, diagnostics and animal models'. China's commitment to rapidly acquiring knowledge about this new virus was a critical factor in enabling the country to contain, suppress and eventually extinguish the epidemic.

Meanwhile, owing to Wuhan's position as a central Chinese transportation hub, the virus was moving globally. Clinicians reported cases in real time as they arrived in Nepal,[9] Canada,[10] Italy,[11] the US[12] and Singapore.[13] The case of Italy was an especially important example of how science could contribute to a more effective national and international response.

During February, it was becoming clear that Italy was facing an outbreak of unusual force. Giuseppe Remuzzi directs the Mario Negri Institute of Pharmacology Research in Bergamo. As he saw his hospital fill with patients requiring intensive care and ventilation, he began to foresee a humanitarian crisis unfolding. By early March, Italy, and especially the Lombardy region in the north, had seen over 12,000 cases of infection, with 827 deaths. The average age of those who had died was 81 years, and more than two-thirds of patients had medical histories of diabetes, cancer or heart disease. Remuzzi calculated that Italian hospitals simply did not have the capacity to treat the mass of patients that would present once the wave of SARS-CoV-2 swept through the country. They predicted that more than 30,000 Italians would be infected by 15 March.[14]

Remuzzi was direct in his conclusions: Italy faced a predicament of 'unmanageable dimensions', one that would have 'catastrophic results'. He predicted that the events that had overwhelmed Hubei would soon engulf Lombardy. The numbers unfortunately support Remuzzi's worst fears. At the time of writing, Italy is third after the US and the UK in its burden of death from COVID-19.

The story of COVID-19 in the US is one of the strangest paradoxes of the whole pandemic. No other country in the world has the concentration of scientific skill, technical knowledge and productive capacity possessed by the US. It is the world's scientific superpower bar none. And yet this colossus of science utterly failed to bring its expertise successfully to bear on the policy and politics of the nation's response. More people died in the US from COVID-19 in three months than during the entire Vietnam War (there were 58,318 US soldiers killed in action in Vietnam between 1955 and 1975; deaths from COVID-19 exceeded that figure on 28 April 2020).

The first case of COVID-19 in the US was reported on 21 January in a young man from Washington state who had returned from Wuhan a week earlier, on 15 January. Nancy Messonnier, who directed America's National Center for Immunization and Respiratory Diseases, called the news 'concerning'.

Commenting on the events unfolding in China, on 24 January President Trump wrote on Twitter that 'It will all turn out well.' Anthony Fauci, the long-standing and much respected director of the National Institute of Allergy and Infectious Diseases, noted, 'We don't want the American public to be worried about this because their risk is low.' But, by 30 January, the US Centers for Disease Control and Prevention reported the country's first case of person-to-person transmission, in a woman whose husband had been in Wuhan. Still, the government assessed the risk to the American public as 'low'.

But by 31 January, the day after WHO declared a PHEIC, President Trump had called coronavirus a public health emergency. Travel bans were implemented. Yet the government still didn't seem to comprehend the urgency of the threat. By 12 February, the first American had died of COVID-19. On 21 February, Messonnier agreed that it was now 'very possible' that spread in the community could take place. By the end of February, that possibility became a reality, and Vice-President Mike Pence was appointed by Trump to lead the nation's response to COVID-19.

Pence and Fauci agreed that testing and isolation of those who tested positive should be the cornerstone of their national strategy. But it became clear during March that America's healthcare system, in Fauci's words, was 'not set up for that'. 'That is a failing,' he said. The result was that by the end of March efforts to contain the virus had floundered.

The US had become the most infected nation on the planet. Social distancing and avoiding mass gatherings now became the approved policy of the Trump administration. But the virus had taken hold and deaths began to escalate – as did unemployment as the economy crashed. By May, the US Treasury had announced it was borrowing a record $3 trillion to pay for the coronavirus relief measures passed by Congress.

Wuhan began its lockdown early – on 23 January. Through strenuous efforts to cut the lines of viral transmission, China was able to begin to lift its restrictions on 8 April. As it did so, Deborah Birx, appointed by Pence as the coordinator of the White House coronavirus task force, reported that the epidemic had now reached its peak in the US. By 11 April, the country had surpassed Italy in its number of COVID-19 deaths. Every state had been affected. As the economy imploded further, and as protests broke out about the stay-at-home orders, President Trump turned his fire on China and WHO. On 14 April, he announced that he would stop funding the agency, and he accused China of withholding crucial information about the virus.

The situation in the UK was no less disastrous. From the last week in January, it took the UK government seven weeks to recognise the seriousness of COVID-19. It wasted the whole of February and most of March, when ministers should have been preparing the country for the arrival of a deadly new virus. Why? Inexplicably, medical and scientific advisers to the UK government ignored the warnings coming from China.

Boris Johnson won a general election on 13 December 2019 on the promise that he would 'get Brexit done'. Britain was leaving the European Union on 31 January, a day, the new prime minister said, that symbolised a moment for 'national renewal and change'. On 26 February, less than a month after WHO had declared a PHEIC, he announced an integrated review of foreign policy, defence, security and international development. Johnson claimed this review would be the largest since the Cold War. He spoke about 'the changing nature of threats we face'. But he failed to mention the new coronavirus seeding itself across the country. Did Brexit influence the UK's go-it-alone approach?

By 2 March, Prime Minister Johnson was chairing COBRA, the civil contingencies committee that is convened to handle issues of national emergency. After that meeting, he agreed that COVID-19 presented 'a significant challenge'. 'But we are well-prepared,' he said. Was Johnson aware of Exercise Cygnus and its clear conclusion in 2016 that the UK was most definitely not well-prepared? If he was, he lied to the public.

If he was not, then he is surely guilty of misconduct in public office. Remember: a pandemic is top of the UK's National Risk Register. A prime minister should reasonably be expected to understand the capability of his country to address the most severe civil emergency risk.

The best that Prime Minster Johnson could do was advise hand-washing. He was still arguing that the UK 'remains extremely well-prepared' on 3 March.

On 5 March, when there were 85 confirmed cases of COVID-19 in the UK, Johnson went on national television to continue to minimise the risks of the virus. On ITV's *This Morning* he said, 'Perhaps you could sort of take it on the chin, take it all in one go and allow the disease, as it were, to move through the population without really taking as many draconian measures. I think we need to strike a balance.' He displayed his own disregard for the risks of infection by regularly shaking hands with those he met – and bragging about it afterwards.

But by 7 March the government was advising people with symptoms to self-isolate. Ministers seemed unsure of what to do. Let the epidemic rip through the population – 'take it on the chin' – or do something more? By 12 March, the UK had stopped its policy of test, contact trace and isolate – a decision later acknowledged as a mistake. For still unknown reasons, the UK government waited. And watched.

The scientists advising ministers seemed to believe that this new virus could be treated much like influenza. Graham Medley, one of the government's expert scientific advisors, was disarmingly explicit. In an interview on the BBC's television programme *Newsnight*, he explained the UK's early attitude – to encourage a controlled epidemic of large numbers of people in order to generate 'herd immunity'. He recommended 'a situation where the majority of the population are immune to the infection. And the only way of developing that, in the absence of a vaccine, is for the majority of the population to become infected.' Medley advocated 'a nice big epidemic'. 'What we are going to have to try and do', he said, was to 'manage this acquisition of herd immunity and minimise the exposure of people who are vulnerable.' Sir Patrick Vallance, the government's chief scientific advisor, suggested that the goal was to infect 60 per cent of the UK's population.

As March proceeded, government ministers became increasingly anxious. But they were still unable to act decisively. Their staccato decision-making suggested an atmosphere of mounting confusion and fear. On 16 March, the public was advised to cease non-essential travel. On 18 March, schools were closed. And on 20 March, entertainment venues, bars and restaurants were shut. It took until 23 March for the 'stay at home' order to be issued. Critical time had been lost.

What is so mysterious is that it didn't need the predictions of scientists at Imperial College London in March to estimate the impact of a 'watch-and-wait' approach. Any numerate school student could make the calculation. With a mortality of 1 per cent among 60 per cent of a UK population of some 66 million people, the UK could expect almost 400,000 deaths. The huge wave of critically ill patients that would result from this strategy of 'take it on the chin' herd immunity would quickly overwhelm the NHS, just as had been the case in Italy. The UK's best scientists had known since the first report from China in January that COVID-19 was a lethal illness. Yet they too did too little, too late.

Remuzzi had also warned European countries. Describing the lessons of his experience in Lombardy, he wrote that 'These considerations might also apply to other European countries that could have similar numbers of patients infected and similar needs regarding intensive care admissions.' And yet the UK continued with its strategy of encouraging the epidemic to tear through communities unchecked.

Nobody can claim ignorance. Nobody can say this interpretation of events is hindsight. Writing in 1994 in her treatise *The Coming Plague*, Laurie Garrett concluded,

> Ultimately, humanity will have to change its perspective on its place in Earth's ecology if the species hopes to stave off or survive the next plague. Rapid globalization of human niches requires that human beings everywhere on the planet go beyond viewing their neighborhoods, provinces, countries, or hemispheres as the sum total of their personal ecospheres. Microbes, and their vectors, recognize none of the artificial boundaries erected by human beings … In the microbial world warfare is a constant … Time is short.[15]

If you think Garrett's language rhetorical hyperbole, consult the more sober analysis from the US Institute of Medicine in 2004. They evaluated the lessons of the 2003 SARS outbreak, quoting Goethe: 'Knowing is not enough; we must apply. Willing is not enough; we must do.' The Institute of Medicine concluded, 'The rapid containment of SARS is a success in public health, but also a warning ... If SARS reoccurs ... health systems worldwide will be put under extreme pressure ... Continued vigilance is vital.'[16] But the world ignored these warnings.

Consider these outbreaks: Hendra in 1994, Nipah in 1998, SARS in 2003, MERS in 2012 and Ebola in 2014. These major human epidemics of viruses that came from animal hosts were a sign. We should probably not be surprised that these signals of threat went unheeded. We are all guilty of confirmation bias – ignoring information that doesn't match our own view or experience of the world. How many of us have experienced a pandemic? Catastrophes reveal the weaknesses of human memory. How can one plan for a random rare event? Surely the sacrifices will be too great? But, as seismologist Lucy Jones argues in *The Big Ones* (2018), 'Natural hazards are inevitable; the disaster is not.'[17]

Risks can be measured and quantified. As Laurie Garrett and the Institute of Medicine showed so clearly, the dangers of a new epidemic have been known and understood since HIV emerged in the 1980s. And what about HIV? 75 million people have been infected with HIV since the start of that epidemic; 32 million people have died. HIV may not have swept through the world with the pace of SARS-CoV-2, but its shadow remains immeasurably greater and should have alerted governments to be ready for an outbreak of a new viral threat.

In times of crisis, public and politicians alike understand-ably turn to experts. On this occasion the experts – scientists who have modelled and simulated our possible futures – made assumptions that turned out to be mistaken. The UK imagined a pandemic in the image of influenza. The influenza virus is not benign. Annual deaths from influenza vary widely, with a recent peak in the UK of 28,330 deaths in 2014/15 and a low of 1,692 deaths in 2018/19. But influenza is not COVID-19.

China, by contrast, was scarred by its experience of SARS. When the government realised that a new SARS virus was circulating, Chinese officials didn't advise hand-washing, a better cough etiquette and the disposal of tissues. They locked down entire cities and turned off the economy. As one former secretary of state for health in England put it to me, our scientists suffered from a 'cognitive bias' towards the milder threat of influenza.

Perhaps that is why the key government committee, the New and Emerging Respiratory Virus Threats Advisory Group (NERVTAG), concluded on 21 February, three weeks after WHO had declared a PHEIC, that, with one exception, they had no objection to Public Health England's 'moderate' risk assessment of the disease threat to the UK population. That was a genuinely fatal error of judgement.

This failure to escalate the risk assessment led to mortal delays in preparing the NHS for the coming wave of infection. The desperate pleas I received during March and April from frontline NHS staff are painful to read. 'Nursing burnout is at an all-time high and a lot of our heroic nursing staff are on the verge of emotional breakdown.' 'It is sickening that this is happening, and that somehow this country thinks it's okay to let some members of staff get sick, get ventilated, or die.' 'I feel like a soldier going to war without a gun.' 'It's suicide.'

The availability of and access to appropriate personal protective equipment has been appallingly bad for many nurses and doctors. Some hospital trusts planned well. But many, maybe most, were unable to provide the necessary safe equipment to their frontline teams.

At every press conference, the government spokesperson always includes the same line – 'We have been following the medical and scientific advice.' It's a good line. And it's partly true. But government knew – Exercise Cygnus – that the NHS was unprepared. Government knew it had failed to build the necessary intensive-care surge capacity to meet the likely patient demand. As one doctor wrote to me: 'It seems that nobody wants to learn from the human tragedy that happened in Italy, China, Spain ... This is really sad ... Doctors and scientists who are not able to learn from one another.'

The scientists and physicians leading the response to the pandemic in the UK said that keeping deaths from COVID-19 to below 20,000 would be a 'good outcome'. That line was breached on 25 April, 'a very sad day for the nation'.

The official government narrative was that the UK's National Health Service had succeeded in coping with the epidemic. Yet that assessment was only true because thousands of planned appointments and elective procedures were cancelled to create the capacity for the succeeding wave of COVID-19 admissions. 33,000 beds were cleared of patients in England alone to provide the space to absorb the expected influx of patients with COVID-19.

Despite the very best efforts of health workers, the NHS certainly did not cope. It was unable to deliver the necessary surge capacity beyond its normal service provision; it failed to implement a test and isolate policy until late in the outbreak; it did not provide adequate supplies of personal protective equipment, leaving health workers on the frontline of the outbreak response vulnerable to infection; and the separation of social care from the NHS left older citizens unprotected in care homes.

One result of the massive displacement of thousands of planned operations, procedures and appointments was the creation of a backlog of work that will only worsen pressures on already stressed hospitals, community and primary care services, and social care. When Jenny Harries, England's deputy chief medical officer, called the UK's state of preparedness an 'international exemplar', most observers were astonished. The UK's response had been slow, complacent and flat-footed. The country was glaringly unprepared.

\*

COVID-19 has revealed the astonishing fragility of our societies, our shared vulnerability. It has revealed our inability to cooperate, to coordinate and to act together. Perhaps we cannot control the natural world after all. Perhaps we are not quite as dominant as we once thought. If COVID-19 eventually imbues human beings with some humility, then possibly we will, after all, be receptive to the lessons of this lethal virus. Or perhaps we will sink back into our culture of complacent exceptionalism and await the next plague that will surely arrive. To go by recent history, that moment will come sooner than we think.

Something went badly wrong in the way many countries handled COVID-19. In the UK, the government had the services of some of the most talented researchers in the world on which to draw. But somehow there was a collective failure to recognise the signals that Chinese and Italian scientists were sending. The UK had the opportunity and the time to learn from the experience of other countries. For reasons that remain not entirely clear, the UK missed those signals and missed those opportunities.

Perhaps it was the regime of science policymaking that had gone wrong. I believe two charges can be fairly made against the current regime with respect to its handling of this pandemic. First, that it was corrupted – the system resulted in an abuse of entrusted power. It was an abuse of power because the system of science policy formation failed to act on clear and unambiguous signals from China that culminated in a PHEIC from WHO on 30 January. When a PHEIC was called, government scientific advisory committees, such as NERVTAG, together with the chief medical officer and chief scientific advisor, should have urgently started asking questions. They should have contacted their counterparts in China and Hong Kong – Bin Cao, George Gao, George Leung – to seek first-hand testimony about what was happening. They should have called WHO's country office in Beijing to understand their assessment of the situation in

Wuhan. If they had done so, our most senior scientific advisors would have heard the same messages so starkly reported in their published papers from January – a pandemic of a bitterly toxic virus was on its way to Europe. The fact that they apparently took none of these actions is what constitutes the abuse of entrusted power.

Second, that it was collusive – scientists and politicians agreed to act together in order to protect the government, to give the illusion that the UK was an 'international exemplar' in preparedness and made the right decisions at the right time, based upon the science. Every day, as the pandemic moved its venomous way through the population, a minister would deliver a press briefing to announce the daily toll of infection and death. He or she would be flanked by a government scientist or medical advisor. When advisors were asked questions, they would speak with one voice in support of government policy. They never deviated from the political scripts they were given. Why was no PPE reaching frontline health workers? Instead of saying honestly that the lessons of Exercise Cygnus had not been acted upon, the scientific or medical advisor would say the government was doing its best. Why was testing capacity so poor? Instead of saying honestly that the government had ignored WHO's recommendation to 'test, test, test', the advisor would say that testing wasn't appropriate for the UK. Why has the government stopped reporting mortality figures for the UK and other countries? Instead of saying honestly that the government found those figures acutely embarrassing, the advisor would say that such comparisons were spurious and, anyway, they were available elsewhere. Advisors became the public relations wing of a government that had failed its people.

*

Is British science really so corrupted and collusive? Is there no alternative to this broken system of obsequious politico-scientific complicity? Yes, there is.

'Is the government's objective to suppress infection or to manage the infection?', asked Sir David King at the first press conference of a newly formed Independent Scientific Advisory Group for Emergencies (SAGE), held in May. The UK now had two SAGEs. The officially constituted SAGE provides scientific advice to support government decision-making during emergencies. It had seen its reputation collapse during the previous three months. Partly, this loss of credibility arose out of the group's unwillingness to be transparent about its participants and its proceedings. At a moment of national emergency, SAGE's pervasive secrecy and deference to ministers simply became unacceptable. The public had a right to know the evidence on which advice was being made to government – advice that was not only protecting lives but also destroying livelihoods. But the official SAGE luxuriated in elite insouciance. It displayed a very British characteristic: the arrogance of exceptionalism. Rarely has a publicly constituted body been so out of touch with the public mood for accountability.

The Independent SAGE published its membership before holding its first meeting. Sir David King was himself once chief scientific advisor to the UK government, the position now occupied by Sir Patrick Vallance. But King had put together a more gender- and ethnically diverse scientific group than the official SAGE – which had the look of a white male club. The new and more independent version of SAGE was also broader in the range of science upon which it drew. Public health was its core, but it also included experts on epidemic modelling, behavioural science and public policy.

This wider intellectual reach made the recommendations of the Independent SAGE more relevant to the UK's predicament. The first meeting was broadcast on YouTube, giving the public full access to the difficult judgements needed to steer the country out of lockdown. It also displayed the challenges faced by political decision-makers who had to ensure the country was prepared should a second wave of the pandemic ensue.

The recommendations from the Independent SAGE focused on five additional areas beyond seeking clarification of the government's overall objective in managing the pandemic. First, how was the government planning to ensure financial security for the most marginalised groups in society, including black and minority ethnic populations (a group that suffered four times the mortality rate from COVID-19)? This virulent coronavirus has revealed, exploited and accentuated deep socio-economic and racial disparities in the UK. As Zubaida Haque noted, the existing 'economic safety net is not enough.' Haque is deputy director of the Runnymede Trust and an expert on race equality. The government had ignored those least able to protect themselves, she argued.

Second, community public health and primary care systems needed to be urgently strengthened. Allyson Pollock is a professor of public health at Newcastle University. She pointed out that community public health had been decimated during the past decade. Third, improved long-term planning was needed to meet the needs of those most at risk of infection – by increasing intensive care capacity, for example. Fourth, policies were needed to control borders – at seaports, at airports and for train services to Europe.

And, finally, the emphasis on vaccines as a means to return life to some measure of normality needed to be tempered by accepting that no vaccine was a going to be a perfect 'magic bullet'. As emphasised by Deenan Pillay, professor of virology at University College London, even if a vaccine was made and manufactured by the end of 2020, it was unlikely to be completely safe and effective, and it would almost certainly not be taken up universally.

King's argument for setting up a rival body to SAGE was that ensuring public trust in the scientific advice given to government demanded that those giving advice should not be dependent on the government.[18] Too many members of the official SAGE were government employees. Astonishingly, the official SAGE allowed the participation of the architect of Brexit, Dominic Cummings, who had been appointed by Prime Minister Boris Johnson as his chief political advisor. The official SAGE was impossibly compromised.

This first meeting of an Independent SAGE set a new standard for science policymaking. The openness of the process, vigour of discussion, and identification of issues barely discussed by politicians injected much needed candour into public and political discussions about COVID-19. It's hard to predict the longevity of this new group. But its point was made. On the same day it held its first meeting, the government published the names of members of the official SAGE.

*

Eventually, some senior scientists found the collusion between science and government impossible to bear. They broke ranks. Nobel laureate Sir Paul Nurse went on the *Today* programme on 22 May to argue that the government was on the 'back foot'. 'Maybe there's a strategy there, I don't see it,' he said. 'We are desperate for clear leadership at all levels.'

*

I sat with the director-general of the WHO in Geneva in February. He was in despair. Dr Tedros had been criticised for not calling a PHEIC sooner. But when he did so, and when he subsequently asked for the modest sum of $675 million to help WHO combat the growing global pandemic, countries ignored his pleas. Most countries eventually took the right actions to extinguish this pandemic. But their governments lost valuable time. There were preventable deaths. The system failed. When we have finally suppressed this outbreak, when life returns to some semblance of normality, difficult questions will have to be asked and answered. Because we can't afford to fail again. We may not have a second chance.

# 4

# First Lines of Defence

An epidemic is a sudden disastrous event in the same way as a hurricane, an earthquake, or a flood. Such events reveal many facets of the societies with which they collide. The stress they cause tests social stability and cohesion.

Dorothy Porter, *Health, Civilization and the State* (1999)

What does it mean to possess a health service? At the very least, it represents the commitment of people living in a society (past and present) to the twin ideas of solidarity and collective action. By solidarity I mean the feelings of empathy and responsibility we all feel and owe towards one another. Solidarity stands in opposition to the principles of individualism and competition which so dominate and shape our lives in twenty-first-century capitalist, and even authoritarian, nation-states.

The existence of, public support for, and continuous development of a health system suggests that we are prepared to make personal material contributions (e.g., through taxation) to institutions that protect and strengthen the lives not only of ourselves but also of others in our society. That willingness to act on behalf of others is the second feature of a health system – our commitment to a belief in our interdependence and reciprocal responsibility towards one another and also to the collective action necessary to make those feelings real and tangible.

The whole basis of our society depends upon these two principles. COVID-19 has tested their resilience. So many people have died, so many families are in mourning, so many communities have been left scarred by disease. We have been shocked by the power of a virus to throw our societies into chaos, to deprive us of our lives and liberties, and to destroy economies. COVID-19 invites us, calls on us, requires us to rethink who we are and what we value.

One fundamental shift in our thinking surely has to be around the concept of our security. Ever since the birth of the nation-state, security has been viewed as the protection of national borders and each country's political sovereignty. An infectious disease such as SARS-CoV-2 transcends states, borders and sovereignty. A virus is not amenable to passport controls or military defeat, despite the frequent invocation of the idea of an 'invisible enemy'. No person, no country, can survive in splendid isolation.

COVID-19 has taught us to reimagine security as being about people and communities, about our survival, our livelihoods and our dignity. Disease is a threat to our human security, and pandemics are the most dangerous threats of all. Pandemics disrupt every part of our society, leaving us wounded and vulnerable. Protecting our security is not only about having strong military defences. Our security also depends on strong social institutions – and an effective health system is the most important defence we have to protect that security. Think of the security of your own family if you do not believe me.

The Chinese government was deeply traumatised by its experience of SARS in 2002–3. China's leaders felt the threat a virus posed to their political model. The acceptance by the Chinese people of a government that restricted political freedoms in return for annual double-digit economic growth was a particular kind of social contract that carried inherent risks. For, if economic growth was endangered, the social contract that enabled the Chinese Communist Party to rule unchallenged would be in danger too. Not since the events of Tiananmen Square on 4 June 1989 has the Chinese regime felt so vulnerable. They understand that national security means health security. And so they were ready.

When SARS-CoV-2 emerged, the first reaction of local officials in Wuhan was to suppress the evidence for its existence. The life of Li Wenliang will forever stand as an example of a courageous commitment to warn his fellow citizens of the impending threat. But once authorities in Beijing – and especially those in the National Health Commission (China's Ministry of Health), the China Center for Disease Control and Prevention and the Chinese Academy of Medical Sciences – learned of what was taking place in Hubei Province, they recognised the threat. If the virus took hold, the government would simultaneously have to cut the lines of viral transmission and protect its health system from being overwhelmed. China's government achieved both objectives through a deceptively simple innovation – the Fangcang shelter hospital.[1]

These vast temporary hospitals, rapidly built in existing stadiums and exhibition halls, were used to isolate patients with COVID-19 from their families and workplaces. They provided food and basic medical care, enabling ongoing illness among those admitted to be monitored carefully. If a patient deteriorated, they could be transferred to a hospital with proper intensive care facilities.

The word 'Fangcang' sounds like 'Noah's Ark' in Chinese. In Wuhan, three of these shelter hospitals were constructed and were ready to accept up to 4,000 patients with mild to moderate disease by early February. A further thirteen similar shelter hospitals were opened in the succeeding weeks, providing 12,000 beds. As the epidemic came under control and subsided, the hospitals were decommissioned, the last being closed by mid-March.

Why admit patients with mild disease to a shelter hospital instead of insisting on home isolation? The reason lay in the way in which the virus was being transmitted. With workplaces and public venues closed, most infections were being spread within families. It was essential to remove anyone who fell ill from a place where further transmission could take place.

Shelter hospitals released pressure from existing healthcare facilities. The approximately 80 per cent of patients with mild to moderate disease could be managed effectively and efficiently in these temporary hospitals, receiving basic medical care and, where necessary, oxygen and intravenous fluids. A patient's temperature, respiratory rate, oxygen saturation and blood pressure were all carefully followed. Mobile diagnostic units gave additional access to imaging and laboratory services. Any worsening of a patient's condition could be detected early, allowing for rapid referral to a hospital with more specialist healthcare facilities.

The organisation of Fangcang shelter hospitals contributed to quickly reducing the reproduction rate, $R_0$, of SARS-CoV-2. They undoubtedly saved lives. The hospitals were staffed with doctors and nurses mobilised from outside Wuhan. As a group of Chinese doctors involved in the organisation and delivery of care to patients with COVID-19 noted, 'By embracing Fangcang shelter hospitals, many countries and communities worldwide could boost their response to the current COVID-19 pandemic as well as future epidemics and disasters.'

Sadly, many countries afflicted by COVID-19 were unable to respond in such agile and creative ways.

*

While the epicentre of the pandemic was Wuhan, the virus quickly spread to other Asian nations. Singapore confirmed its first imported case of COVID-19 on 23 January. Inbound flights to the city-state were banned. Several clusters of disease were identified and close contacts were quarantined.

Hong Kong also followed WHO's recommendation to 'test, test, test'. Those who were found to be positive for coronavirus were quarantined in hospital. Contacts were traced and told to self-isolate. Borders were strictly controlled – anyone arriving from a country with cases of COVID-19 was required to go into quarantine for fourteen days. Quarantine facilities were expanded. Schools were closed and people were encouraged to work from home. No lockdown was formally imposed. Instead, the public voluntarily chose to alter their behaviour, avoid mass gatherings and wear face masks.

The coronavirus arrived in Taiwan on 21 January. By May, according to the Johns Hopkins Coronavirus Resource Center, there had been only 440 confirmed cases of infection and seven deaths. The Taiwanese government's response has been widely praised. The government put the country on high alert in January as the first reports of COVID-19 began to emerge from the Chinese mainland. Those entering Taiwan were screened for infection. After 21 January, Taiwan suspended all air travel to China and quarantined anyone arriving from the mainland. Personal protective equipment was secured, physical distancing implemented, schools closed, quarantine centres established and mask wearing on public transport mandated. Chen Chien-jen, Taiwan's vice-president, is an epidemiologist. His understanding of the threat of this SARS-like pandemic likely made a crucial difference to Taiwan's response. But, because the country's observer status at WHO meetings is blocked by the Chinese government in Beijing, the world will not have a full and complete opportunity to learn from Taiwan's success.

In South Korea, the epidemic took a strange turn. Between 19 January and 18 February, the country reported only thirty cases and no deaths. Patient 31 changed all that. Within ten days there were 2,300 cases. Patient 31 was a super-spreader – a person who passes the virus to a far larger number of people.

She had travelled from Wuhan to Seoul and Daegu, visited a hospital to be treated for a road traffic injury, attended church services (with 1,100 others at the Shincheonji Church of Jesus) and went to a hotel. The government's response was decisive and comprehensive. It had learned lessons from an outbreak of MERS in 2015. A task force was appointed, including all government ministries and regional and city administrations. This emphasis on coordination and transparency worked. The lesson the government learned from MERS was the importance of testing and tracing. They closed schools, but they didn't impose a lockdown. The epidemic peaked on 29 February.

When the virus arrived in Europe, several countries were overwhelmed. Italy suffered nothing less than a humanitarian catastrophe. Spain imposed a full lockdown and a state of emergency on 14 March. But the health system was wholly unprepared, with daily deaths peaking at one point at over 700. Even on 8 March, the government allowed hundreds of thousands of people to take part in nationwide marches for International Women's Day. Health workers had poor access to personal protective equipment, leaving 50,000 infected by May. Ordinary healthcare was disrupted. And care homes became particular points of vulnerability.

In Madrid, a skating rink was commandeered as a temporary emergency morgue. On 9 April, Médecins Sans Frontières issued an urgent alert to the Spanish authorities, warning that older Spanish citizens were dying alone in residential care homes and hospitals without their families. As the epidemic ebbed, it became clear that the Spanish government had badly underestimated how fast the virus could spread and the seriousness of the disease it caused. The first COVID-19 case was reported in Spain on 31 January and the country's first death was on 13 February. And yet politicians, and even scientists, failed to respond to these early warnings.

In France, the outbreak began in early February at about the same time as in South Korea. Jean-Paul Moatti, former director and president of the prestigious French National Research Institute for Sustainable Development, was highly critical of the French government's response. He wrote, 'a South Korean strategy of mass testing, contact tracing, and physical distancing was not adopted in France.' Instead, France imposed a lockdown on 17 March. The country didn't have the laboratory capacity for mass testing, and the government claimed mass testing was not needed anyway. They reversed that position at the end of March. France has the third highest number of deaths from COVID-19 in Europe, after only Italy and Spain.

The COVID-19 outbreak in Germany began with a Chinese woman travelling to Bavaria from Shanghai on 19 January, after having met her parents who had come from Wuhan. By 27 January, the first case of infection was confirmed. A month later, after travel to Wuhan had been restricted, the German government established a crisis management committee. The number of cases continued to rise, reaching over 3,000 by 13 March. Restrictions were imposed the following week, with the closure of schools, clubs and bars. Borders were strengthened. The government banned events with fifty or more people. Churches and shops were next to be closed, on 16 March. On

18 March, Chancellor Angela Merkel said that COVID-19 was Germany's biggest challenge since the Second World War. A 'contact ban' was introduced. Numbers of infections continued to rise, but the pace of that rise began to stabilise. By 3 April, 1,100 Germans had died. By 11 April that figure had more than doubled, to 2,736 deaths. Yet, by 15 April, Merkel was ready to ease restrictions. Some shops and schools began partly to reopen. Germany seemed to have avoided the calamity suffered by its neighbours.

How did Germany escape the fate of the UK, Italy and France? Germany started testing, contact tracing and isolating infected patients early in February. The government recommended physical distancing and a fourteen-day quarantine period faster than most other countries. And Germany's well-funded health system had sufficient capacity to cope. The chancellor, Angela Merkel, a scientist herself, delivered clear and precise public messages. Lines of viral transmission were therefore cut quickly. The country's federal structure may have played a part too. The epidemic was managed locally in communities rather than exclusively from Berlin. Cities established their own testing centres, creating a network of 170 laboratories across the country. Despite these good reasons, Germany's relatively soft landing as it emerged from the pandemic still remains something of an enigma. Will the country be so well-prepared and fortunate if and when a second wave of the virus arrives?

New Zealand was an even more astonishing story of success. This country of 5 million citizens had suffered only 1,147 cases of COVID-19 and 21 deaths by mid-May. Prime Minister Jacinda

Ardern reacted quickly after the first case was reported on 28 February, in a woman who had returned home from Iran, via Indonesia. By 21 March, Ardern had raised the country's alert level and launched a national test, trace and isolate programme. By 23 March, the country had reported 102 cases. That was enough to trigger a lockdown. 'We only have 102 cases', said Ardern, 'but so did Italy once.' She went hard and early. She closed the country's borders. And she called a state of national emergency on 25 March. The epidemic peaked in early April, and by 15 May the country was returning to normal life. Ardern is one of the few political leaders to emerge from the pandemic with her reputation enhanced. She had good fortune on her side. New Zealand is a relatively isolated country with a low population density. But her clear, consistent and confident messaging to the public was a model of political choreography in a crisis.

Sweden was another outlier, but for different reasons. Anders Tegnell, the country's state epidemiologist, has been accused of pursuing a policy of herd immunity, which has led (as of mid-May 2020) to over 33,000 cases of COVID-19 and 3,992 deaths. But that is neither fair nor true. The first case of COVID-19 was diagnosed on 31 January, in a woman returning from Wuhan. Although no national lockdown has been introduced, Tegnell has issued a series of strong recommendations, which most people have complied with – limits on mass gatherings, closure of secondary schools and universities, working from home, avoiding unnecessary travel, and physical distancing. His focus was on individual responsibility rather than political instruction. It was a huge gamble and the backlash is growing.

India appears to have steered an even safer course through the pandemic, despite having a population of 1.4 billion people. The country's first case was reported on 30 January. The government closed its international borders early, and a subsequent lockdown, the largest in the world, was praised by WHO as 'tough and timely'. Lockdown also gave the government time to prepare for the possible surge in cases. Still, India's diverse population, its harsh health inequalities, widening economic and social disparities, and distinct cultural features presented extreme challenges.

Although it is one country, India is in truth a nation of nations – 28 quasi-autonomous states and eight union territories. Important and often impressive differences in preparedness and response emerged at state level. In Kerala, for example, state authorities drew on their experience with an outbreak of Nipah virus in 2018 to use extensive testing, contact-tracing and community mobilisation to contain the virus and maintain a low mortality rate. Odisha's exposure to previous natural disasters meant crisis preparations were already in place and were simply repurposed to address COVID-19. Hospitals dedicated to admitting patients were quickly requisitioned. Maharashtra, which endured the highest number of diagnosed cases, used drones to monitor physical distancing during lockdown and applied a cluster containment strategy to control the disease within a defined geographic area. On identifying three or more COVID-19-positive patients, a 3 kilometre radius around a patient's home was surveyed house to house for fourteen days to detect further cases, contact trace and raise public awareness.

Rajasthan imposed curfews and a ban on spitting. Uttar Pradesh, India's most populous state, expanded its laboratory testing capacity. But, given the country's overall limited testing capacity, a sparse public health workforce and certain challenging disease characteristics, including mild and asymptomatic cases and rapid spread, it is unlikely that states were able to reach the levels of operational excellence needed to control the outbreak fully. Nevertheless, there was an extraordinary response from sections of civil society. To fight fake news about the pandemic, the Indian Scientists' Response to COVID-19 became a grassroots initiative to neutralise disinformation. States deserve much of the credit for the country's partly successful response. There were important lessons for other countries to learn from India.

One shortcoming of India's COVID-19 response was the low rate of testing. Another constraint was an acute shortage of health workers, while yet another consisted of the large communities living in slums with no possibility for physical distancing. The government's sudden enforcement of lockdown also disadvantaged already vulnerable populations. There was a mass exodus of migrant workers, and concerns rose about starvation among those who worked in the informal economy. Implementing public health measures is always difficult in places with overcrowded living conditions and inadequate hygiene and sanitation. Non-COVID-19 health services have been disrupted. The pandemic was also used to fan anti-Muslim sentiment and violence after a gathering linked to the group Tablighi Jamaat was identified as the source of a large cluster of cases. Yet India's relatively young population – two-thirds are under 35 years of age – may well have protected the country from a much more severe health crisis.

As for the US, pictures of makeshift mass graves in New York state being dug and filled with wooden coffins taken from refrigerated trucks by prisoners wearing hazmat suits perhaps best summed up the lamentable response by President Trump's administration. His suggestion that patients with COVID-19 might benefit from injections of disinfectant, made at a press conference on 24 April, defined the farce that the American political response became. By May, President Trump was describing the 'attack' of COVID-19 as being worse than Pearl Harbor and 9/11. The US response has been as pitiful as it has been surprising. Opinion polls put only Boris Johnson and Xi Jinping below President Trump in terms of trust. A superpower – or its reputation at least – had been slain by a virus.

Elsewhere, there was chaos. Brazil's President Jair Bolsonaro responded to a question about rapidly rising numbers of COVID-19 cases by saying, 'So what? What do you want me to do?' In Russia, President Putin faced an economic crisis that threatened the stability of his government. He was forced to cancel 9 May Victory Day celebrations that would have triumphantly marked his amendment to the constitution designed to keep him in office until 2036.

\*

One important consequence of the COVID-19 health emergency was the focus it put on the most vulnerable individuals and communities in our society. In the UK, for example, 1.3 million people were 'shielded'. This group included those who had undergone an organ transplant, patients with specific types of cancer and who were undergoing treatment with chemotherapy or radiotherapy, people with severe respiratory disease, those with rarer diseases who were more at risk from infection, and women who were pregnant. They were advised to stay isolated and avoid any face-to-face contact for at least three months.

But just who should be defined as 'vulnerable'? Some critics argued that the definition of those at risk should have been far more capacious. It was known, for example, that older patients had a higher risk of complications and death from COVID-19. Across the UK population, there were 5.7 million people over the age of 70 years. Surely they were vulnerable too. The epidemiology of deaths from COVID-19 also showed a clear relation between having an underlying health condition and death. An additional 2.7 million people under the age of 70 years lived with a condition such as heart disease or diabetes. The total number of vulnerable people in the UK was therefore much higher – 8.4 million people.[2] And what about those who were living in care homes, the homeless, those in prison, or people who lived with severe mental health problems? They were excluded from the government's gaze.

If the NHS has faced its most serious emergency since it was founded in 1948, then the social care system underwent nothing less than devastation – which took place without any politician seeming to know or understand what was happening. But by the end of April the scale of the social care tragedy had become all too clear.

On 28 April, the Office for National Statistics reported that, up to 17 April, 2,906 people had died in care homes from COVID-19-related causes. Additional data showed that, between 18 and 24 April, there had been a further 2,375 COVID-related deaths in social care settings. In total, from 10 to 24 April, 4,343 people had died in residential care and nursing homes from the direct effects of the pandemic. Whereas hospital deaths peaked around 10 April and were now seeing a slow decline, the epidemic raging through care homes was only just beginning. One of the lasting legacies of COVID-19 will be the silent human destruction it wreaked on the most unprotected older members of society.

Black and Asian men and women were four times more likely to die from COVID-19 compared with their white counterparts. This additional risk in particular ethnic communities intersected with pre-existing inequalities in society. After taking account of age and other socio-economic characteristics, the risk of a COVID-19-related death for men and women of black ethnicity reduced to two times more likely than among those of white ethnicity. The Office for National Statistics concluded that 'the difference between ethnic groups in COVID-19 mortality is partly a result of socio-economic disadvantage and other circumstances, but a remaining part of the difference has not yet been explained.' Almost two-thirds of health workers who have died were from an ethnic minority. The UK government has established an inquiry to understand why black and minority ethnic communities are in special jeopardy.

Every government that put its population into lockdown adopted a similar message – stay at home. But that message may have backfired. People did stay at home, even when they had symptoms of life-threatening illness, such as a heart attack, stroke or cancer. The true toll of death from the pandemic will have to include those who didn't receive the emergency care they so urgently needed. The shadow of the pandemic on society will be long and dark.

Health workers were shockingly unprotected. No other group in society was at more immediate risk than those whose job it was to care for people with COVID-19. And yet in many countries they were the least protected. WHO had recommended high standards for the personal protective equipment that should have been available to health workers – a full body gown, a fit-tested mask and visor, and rubber gloves. And yet in many countries all that was available were thin plastic aprons that left arms and legs exposed, inadequate surgical masks, and rubber gloves that left arms vulnerable.

Health workers were left unprotected because governments had failed to procure sufficient supplies of protective equipment as soon as a PHEIC had been declared. It was a stunning act of administrative omission and certainly cost the lives of dozens of health workers in some of the most affected countries. At daily 10 Downing Street press briefings, government ministers would claim that personal protective equipment was being delivered to the frontlines of care and that health workers were safe. At best, these statements turned out to be overpromises. At worst, they were bare-faced lies.

As the epidemic in the UK took hold during March, I received hundreds of messages from health workers on the frontlines of care in the NHS, a collective cry of anguish about their abandonment by government. Their testimonies should be read and remembered: our government deserted the nation's most precious line of human defence.

'It's terrifying for staff at the moment. Still no access to PPE [personal protective equipment] or testing.'

'The situation is horrendous for everyone.'

'There's been no guidelines, it's chaos.'

'I don't feel safe. I don't feel protected.'

'We are literally making this up as we go along.'

'It feels as if we are actively harming patients.'

'We need protection.'

'Total carnage.'

'Humanitarian crisis.'

'Forget lockdown. We are going into meltdown at many practices.'

'The hospitals in London are overwhelmed.'

'The public and media are not aware that today we no longer live in a city with a properly functioning Western healthcare system.'

'How will we protect our patients and staff? I am speechless. It is utterly unconscionable. How can we do this? It is criminal. We feel completely helpless.'

'Brutal on the ground.'

'The tsunami is coming.'

'The situation is dire.'

'It is a national scandal.'

'There is serious failure of leadership.'

'There is a huge staffing crisis.'

'WHO PPE standards are not followed.'

'When generals have lost wars (lives) they have been tried
for treason. What is the appropriate response in our
circumstances?'

'We feel completely abandoned.'

'We feel it's a completely negligent approach and not safe at all.'

'I can't tell you how distraught we feel. It's beyond words.'

'Is anybody actually listening to the concerns and acting?'

'We have been so disappointed with the UK's late response.'

'This is playing with lives.'

'Inadequate PPE, no scrubs, not testing staff.'

'Totally inadequate PPE. No N95 masks. Being sent like lambs to
the slaughter.'

'Today was shambolic in terms of PPE.'

'Sleepwalking into this totally unequipped and unprepared when
we had the luxury of two months to prepare.'

'Patients are now dying of perfectly treatable conditions.'

'Seeing patients with no gowns or goggles.'

'It seems that nobody wants to learn from the human tragedy that
happened in Italy, China, Spain.'

'Ongoing rationing and denying staff access to PPE.'

'Things on the frontline are getting worse, not better.'

'There is a huge mismatch about how the situation is presented
publicly and the reality.'

'Colleagues have to attend disciplinary meetings for speaking
out ... I never thought I lived in a country where freedom of
speech is discouraged.'

*

During the pandemic, UK government ministers encouraged
the public to stand outside their homes every Thursday evening
at 8 pm to 'clap for carers'. This display of support for frontline
health workers was a moving mass public tribute to those who
were risking and sacrificing their lives every day in settings
of acute danger. But the government's injunction to celebrate
carers was tinged with hypocrisy.

One doctor who died on the frontlines of COVID-19 care was
Dr Abdul Mabud Chowdhury. He was a 53-year-old consultant
urologist who worked at the Homerton Hospital in London. He
had appealed to the government for 'appropriate PPE' to 'protect ourselves and our families', and he died of COVID-19 at the
peak of the epidemic in London. His son, Intisar Chowdhury,
has asked the government for a public apology for its failures to
protect health workers from infection. So far, the government
has provided no such apology. The closest it came was a comment by the home secretary, Priti Patel: 'Sorry to anyone who
feels they had not had enough protection.' Intisar Chowdhury
spoke for many health workers when he pointed out that 'Priti
Patel's apology is not a real apology.'

*

Western countries spend a large proportion of their wealth on health. They have highly sophisticated health systems. And they have an extremely well-educated health workforce. One might wonder why the medical leaders in these countries did not do more to alert their governments in January to the impending catastrophe that was about to befall their populations.

In the UK, we have the medical Royal Colleges, the Academy of Medical Sciences, the British Medical Association, Public Health England, the Faculty of Public Health and an array of health think tanks, such as the King's Fund and Nuffield Trust. Yet none reinforced the urgent call to action in early February after WHO declared a PHEIC. That declaration fell on deaf ears within what one might call Britain's 'medical establishment'. Why?

I don't have an answer to this question. I don't believe there was a conspiracy of silence. But there was silence nonetheless. Perhaps the leaders of these bodies, all distinguished scientists and physicians, didn't read the reports coming out of China. Or perhaps they did, but didn't appreciate their importance. Perhaps they didn't understand what a PHEIC meant. Perhaps they understood exactly what was happening but didn't want to criticise government publicly for fear of losing their seat of influence at the political table.

Whatever the reasons, the leadership of medicine in the UK and in many other Western nations let down those they were supposed to protect. They let down the old, the sick and the vulnerable. They betrayed the very people who had invested their trust – and their taxes – in modern medicine. It was a grubby betrayal, a stain on the leadership of a profession whose frontline workers had given so much.

Part of the answer to these systemic failures may lie in a new idea to enter the lexicon of health – the resilient health system.

After the West African Ebola virus disease outbreak of 2015, politicians and policymakers understood the need to build health services that could absorb, withstand and learn from external shocks while retaining their fundamental functions and adapting and transforming to soften the impacts of future shocks. The idea of resilience is still only that – an idea. What does a resilient health system or resilient health service mean in practice? There are some obvious headline elements: adequate financing; a sufficiently large and skilled health workforce; accurate information to guide a response; transparent and accountable leadership; good supplies of essential medicines and health technologies; and the surge capacity to provide additional health services when needed while maintaining everyday clinical care.

One lesson of COVID-19 is that every country must now begin a national conversation about how far it is willing to go – and how much the public is willing to pay – for a health system that can save lives when a pandemic arrives again. As it surely will.

# The Politics of COVID-19

... health professionals of the 21st century will find that they have entered what must become politicised professions. There is nowhere else to go.

Julian Tudor Hart, *The Political Economy of Health Care* (2006)

The response of governments to COVID-19 represents the greatest political failure of Western democracies since the Second World War. A government's first responsibility is its duty of care to citizens. Early government inaction led to the avoidable deaths of thousands of those citizens.

The failures were legion. First, there was a failure of technical advice. Despite possessing some of the world's most talented scientists, nations such as the US, Italy, Spain, France and the UK were unable to harness their knowledge and skills to deliver timely recommendations to forestall the terrifying human impacts of the pandemic.

Partly, this failure was because of a cognitive bias. The expectation in the Western world was that the next infectious pandemic was likely to be a new strain of influenza. The idea that a more severe SARS-like virus might strike was not taken seriously. The relatively small number of scientists advising government existed in groups that did not explicitly consider alternatives to their dominant expectation – they suffered from a disabling 'group think'. Did those scientists read and take seriously the early reports of COVID-19 coming from China, reports that clearly and unambiguously warned of the clinical severity and pandemic potential of the new virus? Did they seek guidance from doctors and scientists in countries that first experienced the effects of COVID-19? If not, why not?

Second, there was a failure of the political process after receiving advice from scientists. During the outbreak, governments repeatedly claimed that they were 'following the science'. But the task of politicians is not merely to accept the advice they are given. They have an obligation to probe, to analyse and to question. Scientists advise, ministers decide. By not doing so, or at least by not doing so to any significant degree, politicians allowed themselves to believe that the pandemic could be withstood and contained without more urgent action.

Third, there were egregious failures of political leadership. Countries failed to establish teams that could develop a vision and a set of values for managing the pandemic. They failed to build trust and confidence among their publics. They failed to act decisively. And they failed to listen, to show humility and to learn from failure.

Fourth, there were catastrophic failures of preparedness. Despite the evidence from Wuhan, political leaders failed to acquire the necessary supplies of personal protective equipment, failed to construct necessary surge diagnostic and clinical capacities, and failed to protect other health services so that usual care could still be offered to those who needed it.

Fifth, there were failures of implementation. Countries often could not expand services to the scale needed in the time available. From testing and tracing to access to ventilators, political leaders struggled to keep ahead of the advancing waves of viral infection. This failure left them unable to manage the response to COVID-19 effectively as the pandemic ensued. It left them unable to plan properly for their lockdown exit strategies.

And, finally, there were serious failures of communication. The messages delivered to the public were often too little, too late. Advice was sometimes confused, contradictory or just plain misleading. When President Trump mused about the possible efficacy of ultraviolet light and disinfectants for preventing and treating COVID-19, he displayed astonishing irresponsibility at a time of national emergency.

Together, these failures constituted an extreme example of state negligence – a failure of governments to exercise their duty of care by ignoring evidence of possible danger, thereby exposing people to the risk of severe, sometimes fatal, harm. The evidence shows that governments could reasonably have been expected to know the risks posed by this new virus. They could reasonably have been expected to implement precautions to have diminished those risks. It was within the power of governments to have prevented this human crisis. They failed to prevent. They omitted to save. Their peoples were abandoned at a moment of spectacular vulnerability. Governments were causally complicit and responsible for these failures.

This message of gross incompetence is not welcome in Western political, medical or even media circles. It conflicts with a geopolitical narrative that casts China as a negative and destructive influence in international affairs. Instead, the preference has been to blame China and WHO. The claim is that China hid the fact of COVID-19. The claim is that WHO colluded with China in a cover-up of enormous proportions.

In April, President Trump initiated 'serious investigations' into China's handling of the COVID-19 outbreak. 'We are not happy with China,' he said on 27 April. 'We believe [the virus] could have been stopped at the source and it wouldn't have spread all over the world.' He called on the Chinese government to be held accountable for its errors, and he threatened to seek financial compensation from Beijing.

There are many reasons to be critical of contemporary China – repression of free speech; imprisonment of dissidents; human rights abuses in Tibet and Xinjiang. But one should perhaps try to put oneself in the position of Chinese policymakers. The common Western narrative about China is that, as the country's economy has grown, so have its strategic political, economic and military ambitions. China, led by an authoritarian Chinese Communist Party, now represents a threat to Western leadership in the free world. The evidence is surely all too clear – China's Belt and Road Initiative, its increasingly aggressive stance on Hong Kong and Taiwan, and its claims over islands in the South China Sea. China has to be contained.

The Chinese perspective is very different. After a century of humiliation at the hands of a colonially minded West, China, proud of its 5,000-year-old civilisation, finally achieved independence in 1949. The country grew erratically and with terrifying mistakes under Mao Zedong, but he at least succeeded in establishing secure national borders. Deng Xiaoping created the conditions for economic expansion, lifting as many as 800 million people out of poverty. The task for every Chinese leader today is to protect the territorial independence and integrity won by Mao and the economic security achieved by Deng. As China advances, so there is more and more to protect. Many of China's policymakers will argue that the government's actions should be seen not as aggressive, but as defensive.

In the case of COVID-19, China's scientists and physicians acted decisively and responsibly to protect the health of the Chinese people within this historical context. They warned their government, their government warned WHO, and WHO warned the world. Western democracies failed to listen to those warnings. There are questions for both the Chinese government and WHO to answer. But to blame China and WHO for this global pandemic is to rewrite the history of COVID-19 and to marginalise the failings of Western nations.

\*

It is understandable that Western countries would prefer to diminish their own responsibilities. Their governments are facing difficult questions about what they knew and when they knew it. And they are facing their own crises of trust. Polling during the outbreaks consistently showed disapproval over the responses of Western governments. At the peak of the epidemic in the UK, for example, polls showed disapproval rates rising and a fall in confidence that the government had acted quickly enough. Governments needed a new line of defence. And attack, they believed, was the best form of defence.

Placing responsibility for the pandemic on a country already distrusted by many citizens and an international agency that most people had barely heard of were easy diversions. And it seemed to work. Anti-China sentiment grew. And, although WHO received support from many European capitals after President Trump's decision to withdraw funding from the agency, there was little direct opposition to the US government's aggressive stance. After the SARS outbreak in 2002–3, WHO's prestige and influence had never been greater. After COVID-19, its reputation had never been in more jeopardy.

Multilateralism was once again the victim, bloodied and wounded in a geopolitical war of words. Great power rivalry was ushering in a second Cold War, which dominated and shaped the international response to COVID-19. Globalism, international solidarity and cooperation between states were sacrificed in favour of unilateralism, nationalism and populist self-interest. It was a sad and disappointing contrast to the unanimity among nations following the SARS outbreak in 2002–3.

The war against WHO was an unexpected twist in the story of COVID-19. As the world's only global health agency, WHO tries hard to be strictly apolitical, often to the frustration of its partners and supporters in civil society who want it to flex its political muscles more readily. Its dependency on budget contributions from its member states means that the agency is exquisitely sensitive to criticism from those same member states. To retain continued financial backing, each director-general must work hard to keep its richest donors happy.

When I first began visiting WHO's headquarters in Geneva in the 1990s, senior officials repeatedly reminded me that a quarter of their budget came from the US government. Whatever WHO said or did always had to be reflected through the prism of US interests. And yet during COVID-19, and despite close collaboration between WHO scientists and technical specialists at the CDC in Atlanta, WHO became one of the chief targets of the US administration. The attack by President Trump, accusing the organisation of being 'China-centric', became an unrivalled moment of vulnerability in the agency's 72-year history.

Dr Tedros sought to fight back, as diplomatically as he could –

The United States of America has been a longstanding and generous friend to WHO, and we hope it will continue to be so. We regret the decision of the President of the United States to order a halt in funding to the World Health Organization. With support from the people and government of the United States, WHO works to improve the health of many of the world's poorest and most vulnerable people ... WHO is reviewing the impact on our work of any withdrawal of US funding and we will work with our partners to fill any financial gaps we face and to ensure our work continues uninterrupted.

But the political rift was deep, the partnership broken. Republican congressional members backed President Trump. The chairman of the Senate Finance Committee, Chuck Grassley, accused WHO of being 'slow to raise the global alarm' about the new coronavirus. In a letter to Dr Tedros, Grassley wrote that, 'Unfortunately, there is ample reason to question WHO's response to early signs of this outbreak in China. The lack of independent analysis and advice in the face of initial misleading public messaging from China has resulted in several countries scrambling to make up for lost time.'

When challenged about his decision, President Trump doubled down: 'They called it wrong. They call it wrong. They really, they missed the call.' A group of congressional Republicans signed a letter calling on Dr Tedros to resign before US funding was restored.

All who know WHO know that the agency is an imperfect institution. It is a bureaucracy that puts process before action, diplomacy before advocacy, and compromise before perseverance. WHO is a creature of its member states, reflecting their weaknesses, defects and frailties. Every new director-general pledges to reform WHO, and every director-general stumbles amid its glutinous protocols. But WHO serves a vital role. It gathers the world's best scientists to set standards for health, standards that countries use to advance the wellbeing of their peoples. In the poorest nations of the world, WHO provides indispensable support to ministries of health, health services and health workers.

The world needs a strong WHO to protect the human and

health security of the world's poorest peoples, and the world needs a strong US government to support it both financially and politically. The sudden collapse of US backing for the organisation is a severe setback for global health security. The relationship between WHO and the US government is unlikely to be healed while both Dr Tedros and President Trump remain in their positions. One or both will almost certainly have to depart their roles before relations can be restored.

\*

I have already discussed the many strange stories of disinformation – the infodemic – that emerged during the crisis of COVID-19. What was even more surprising and unexpected was that governments themselves resorted to political disinformation campaigns in order to defend their own roles in managing the outbreak. These efforts to rewrite the narrative of COVID-19 are important to document. Just as there has been a struggle to contain the outbreak, so there is a struggle to control the way the public views government management of the outbreak.

In the UK, for example, ministers have claimed they did not pursue a policy of herd immunity early in the epidemic. The statements from politicians and science advisors clearly prove the opposite. Ministers argue that they have always supported testing for the virus. On the contrary, Jenny Harries, the deputy chief medical officer, made clear that testing was not appropriate for the UK. Ministers say that they have always prioritised the protection of older people living in care homes. The figures for deaths in care homes show otherwise. The constantly repeated message of 'stay at home – protect the NHS – save lives' suggested that protecting the public has been the overriding objective of the UK government. In fact, that message became official government policy only when Prime Minister Boris Johnson spoke to the nation on 23 March instructing people to stay at home. And then there was the statement that the UK was an 'international exemplar' in pandemic preparedness. The numbing toll of deaths displays the complete deceit of that claim.

I became entangled in one effort to manipulate the government's message to its advantage. On 19 April, the *Sunday Times* Insight team published a detailed analysis entitled, 'Coronavirus: 38 days when Britain sleepwalked into disaster'. The central thesis of the article was one that I had articulated in evidence to the House of Commons Select Committee on Science and Technology on 25 March – namely, that the government had wasted February and early March when it should have prepared for the arrival of the pandemic into the UK. The *Sunday Times* wrote, 'The government ignored warnings from scientists and lost a crucial five weeks in the fight to tackle the coronavirus, despite being in a perilously poor state of preparation for a pandemic.'

That same weekend, the government put out a long rebuttal, in which they wrote:

The editor of the Lancet, on exactly the same day – 23 January – called for 'caution' and accused the media of 'escalating anxiety' by talking of a 'killer virus' and 'growing fears'. He wrote: 'In truth, from what we currently know, 2019-nCoV has moderate trans-missibility and relatively low pathogenicity. There is no reason to foster panic with exaggerated language.' The Sunday Times is suggesting that there was a scientific consensus around the fact that this was going to be a pandemic – that is plainly untrue.

This government statement was an extraordinary twisting of the truth, Kremlinesque in its audacity. My tweet, sent on 24 January, was commenting on lurid newspaper headlines that did indeed risk fostering panic. Panic is never a good public health strategy. Instead, what was needed was a careful and thoughtful discussion of the evidence from China and what it meant for the UK.

Later that same day, 24 January, I tweeted a link to the first paper *The Lancet* published describing the seriousness of the clinical presentation of COVID-19. I sent a second tweet with a link to a second paper published that day proving per-son-to-person transmission. In a further tweet I called what was taking place in Wuhan 'A novel coronavirus outbreak of global health concern'. The next day, 25 January, I drew attention to the issue of intensive care capacity and asked why there had as yet been no discussion of what was clearly an urgent clinical challenge: 'A third of patients so far have required admission to ICU … Few countries have the clinical capacity to handle this volume of acutely ill patients. Yet no discussion.'

On 26 January, I tweeted, 'It's now imperative to recall WHO's IHR Emergency Committee to review once again the evidence for and against declaring a Public Health Emergency of International Concern. The needle is moving towards the affirmative.' On 30 January, the director-general of WHO did indeed declare a PHEIC. The facts were utterly opposite to the message from 10 Downing Street. There was an international scientific consensus. The government had simply chosen to ignore it.

In Jacques Ellul's study of the techniques used to manipulate the truth, *Propaganda*, he writes, 'Extreme propaganda must win over the adversary and at least use him by integrating him into its own frame of reference.'[1] The machine of government disinformation was perfectly proving Ellul's disturbing observation. On 10 May, Prime Minister Boris Johnson spoke to the nation. He said of COVID-19, 'We didn't fully understand its effects.' His plaintive excuse will likely become the core defence of his government in the subsequent public inquiry into why the UK failed so spectacularly to protect its citizens. It is a defence that can be and must be refuted.

*

COVID-19 is not a crisis about health. It is something much worse.

Every evening during the peak of the pandemic in the UK, citizens could scour graphs presented by medical and scientific advisors at a daily government press briefing. Was the pandemic advancing or in retreat? New cases of COVID-19. People in hospital with COVID-19. Critical care beds with

COVID-19 patients. Daily COVID-19 deaths in hospital. And then the final and bluntly worded 'global death comparison' – a graph that government scientists actively or passively censored in May as mounting mortality began to embarrass their hitherto crass confidence.

Those with responsibility for leading us through this emergency have called it 'a once in a century global health crisis'. This statement is incorrect on at least two grounds. First, because we cannot know what the rest of the century will bring. It is highly probable that the pandemic of SARS-CoV-2 will be neither the last nor the worst global health crisis of the present century. But, second, and more importantly, this global calamity is not a crisis concerning health. It is a crisis about life itself. We have been tempted in recent years to assume the omnipotence of our species. The idea of the Anthropocene places human activity as the dominant influence on the future for life on our planet. Although this newest of geological eras is supposed to underline the harm our species is doing to fragile planetary systems, paradoxically it also asserts our supremacy. SARS-CoV-2 has revealed the hubris of this view. Our species has many reasons to be self-critical about the effects of our way of life on planetary sustainability. But we are only one species among many, and we are certainly not a dominant influence when faced with a virus that can destroy life with such ease and facility.

If this pandemic is a crisis about life itself, what tentative conclusions might we draw from the effects of COVID-19 so far on human society?

Some clues will be found in the work of Didier Fassin, who studied medicine in Paris before turning to public health and anthropology. Fassin's starting point is the awareness we must all have for the unequal lives we see around us every day. That observation must surely invite us to reflect on the value our society attaches to each human life. We live in a moral economy as well as a market economy. That moral economy is concerned with 'the production, circulation, appropriation, and contestation of values as well as affects around ... life'.[2] What are those values?

In trying to answer that question we somehow have to reconcile 'life as a fact of nature and as a fact of experience'. We can view COVID-19 as a biological challenge to understand, treat and prevent. But we should also understand it as a biographical event in the lives of millions of people. And this is where disease makes its entrance. 'Sickness', Fassin writes, 'sits at the meeting point of biology and biography.' Fassin divides his inquiry into inequality in three parts.

First, he identifies forms of life, by which he means 'ways of being in the world'. The daily insecurities faced by so many citizens draw attention to 'the predicament of contemporary democracies, incapable of living up to the principles that constitute the foundation of their very existence.' The vulnerabilities and precariousness of lives are both universal facts and particular experiences.

Second, he points to an ethics of life. He contrasts the rising legitimacy of those who have a biologically defined and 'empirically robust' proof of disease with the declining legitimacy of lives lived in a particular social setting (such as one of poverty). The physical has prevailed over the political. Fassin calls this ethical trend one of 'biolegitimacy' – a legitimacy of life defined only in biological terms. Life is reduced purely to its physical expression. There is no room for understanding the political conditions within which a life exists. There is no possibility of mobilising public sentiment to defend threats to political lives – lives marked, for example, by inequality. The physical life is legitimate. The political life is not. SARS-CoV-2 preferentially afflicts those who are more vulnerable, less well rewarded and more invisible to those with power.

Third, Fassin focuses on the politics of life, the government of populations, and the effects of politics on human lives. He is interested in how the actions of political regimes differentially influence human lives and reinforce the unequal worth of some of those lives in society. The 'politics of life', he writes, 'are always politics of inequality.'

So what must we say about the politics of COVID-19? We must say, I think, that it is our task to uncover the biographies of those who have lived and died with COVID-19. It is our task to resist the biologicalisation of this disease and instead to insist on a social and political critique. It is our task to understand what this disease means to the lives of those it has afflicted and to use that understanding not only to change our perspective on the world but also to change the world itself. As Fassin himself concludes, our 'critique does not have to choose between militancy and lucidity.'

# The Risk Society Revisited

It is obvious that, in all these instances, the more constantly the persons to be inspected are under the eyes of the persons who should inspect them, the more perfectly will the purpose of the establishment have been attained.

Jeremy Bentham, *Panopticon; or The Inspection House* (1787)

As the number of confirmed cases of COVID-19 in the US soared past 1 million at the beginning of May – with over 64,000 deaths – President Trump was clear about where the blame should be put. On China. The US administration, after decades of confidence-building between the two nations, began a programme of systematic disengagement with its most important strategic competitor. Business, financial and scientific ties started to be severed. The president instructed his intelligence agencies to continue to search for evidence that the pandemic had its origins in a deliberate or accidental leak from a laboratory in Wuhan. Trump claimed to have already seen such evidence, although none has been published and all reputable authorities have dismissed the idea.

The information war launched by the American government included threats to sue China for reparations, block the entry of Chinese telecommunications companies into US markets, and slow American investment into the country. Diplomatic relations between the world's two superpowers stood at an all-time low.

And the fallout from the strained relationship between presidents Trump and Xi Jinping cast a shadow over other institutions critical to the control of the pandemic, notably WHO. On 1 May, as President Trump mused on the origins of the virus, he said, 'I think that the World Health Organization should be ashamed of themselves because they're like the public relations agency for China.' He saw WHO as complicit in a cover-up whose consequences had engulfed the world in a global crisis.

At such points of political stress, mistrust and suspicion, one might step back to investigate some of the possible reasons for this new moment of instability in international relations and what that instability might mean for our collective future.

In his book *Risk Society*, originally published in 1986, Ulrich Beck argued that the creation of wealth in modern societies was always accompanied by the production of new risks. From the climate crisis to increasing inequality, from cyberattacks to environmental pollution, from biodiversity loss to weapons of mass destruction, we see the truth of Beck's claim in our everyday lives. The emergence of new viruses amid the sprawling cities of rapidly advancing nations is another such risk. Beck sought to prove that our world had become 'reflexive' – many of the problems we face today have been generated by ourselves:

While all earlier cultures and phases of social development confronted threats in various ways, society today is *confronted by itself* through its dealings with risks. Risks are the reflection of human actions and omissions, the expression of highly developed productive forces. That means that the sources of danger are no longer ignorance but *knowledge*; not a deficient but a perfected mastery over nature; not that which eludes the human grasp but the system of norms and objective constraints established with the industrial epoch.[1]

Beck was especially critical of 'techno-scientific rationality'. He saw modern science as unable to address the 'growing risks and threats from civilization'. He did not blame individual scientists. Instead, he placed responsibility on 'the institutional and methodological approach of the sciences to risks'. He noted that, 'As they are constituted – with their overspecialized division of labor, their concentration on methodology and theory, their externally determined abstinence from practice – the sciences are *entirely incapable* of reacting adequately to civilizational risks.'[2]

These words seem strikingly apposite for understanding what went wrong in the Western response to the SARS-CoV-2 pandemic. The risks we faced, and continue to face, are not only from a new virus. Those risks are also embedded in the systems we have created and put in place to review and adjudicate on the threat of pandemics – the regime of science policymaking.

What constitutes knowledge about a risk, the assumptions we make about that risk, which evidence is ruled in and out of scope for consideration, who is invited to the table to discuss risks, and what type of science is used to shape advice to politicians – these were all weaknesses within the UK's SAGE and similar bodies in other Western nations. SAGE did not consider the research published at the end of January which set out the magnitude of the threat emerging from Wuhan. It assumed that the most likely danger was a new strain of influenza, not another SARS-like virus. SAGE did not reach out to those with first-hand experience of what was taking place in China. And it did not include experts in intensive care medicine and respiratory medicine, experts who could have better interpreted the evidence from China.

As the epidemic unfolded, it became clear that risk was not evenly distributed across societies. In the UK, for example, the Office for National Statistics examined deaths from COVID-19 according to levels of socio-economic deprivation. The mortality rate of those with COVID-19 in the most deprived areas of England was more than double the rate in the least deprived areas – 55 deaths per 100,000 population compared with 25 deaths per 100,000. Inequality fuelled the accumulating toll of death. COVID-19 has only amplified long-standing inequalities.

Scientific advice and the political reaction to that advice failed to protect the most vulnerable people in our communities. It is here that presidents and prime ministers should look for answers.

There are also questions to be asked about the international response. WHO moved quickly to declare a PHEIC. Daily press briefings and situation reports kept the world informed about the evolution of the pandemic. But, looking back, I think WHO could and should have done more. For example, why didn't the organisation convene nations at an emergency COVID-19 summit immediately after it had declared a PHEIC? By doing so, it could have initiated and led a coordinated global response, pooled evidence and experience, and mobilised and motivated nations to act quickly and decisively. WHO did none of those things. It absented itself from its global leadership role, leaving countries to struggle to respond to COVID-19 alone.

\*

One of the lessons of the SARS epidemic in 2002–3 was the urgent need for better surveillance of new and emerging infectious diseases. It was thanks to surveillance that up-to-date news of the spread of SARS around the world prevented a truly global pandemic. But serious weaknesses in global surveillance efforts were also identified in the aftermath of that near miss. The systems of surveillance present in 2002–3 were not tuned to look for novel threats. There was little collaboration or coordination between countries. The need for continued and strengthened surveillance was clearly evident if a future pandemic was to be prevented.

The goal of the International Health Regulations (IHR), a set of legally binding rules on all countries, is the control of infectious diseases. The regulations exist to manage new infectious disease risks that human societies create. They were first adopted in 1951 as the International Sanitary Regulations and concerned only six diseases – plague, cholera, typhus, relapsing fever, smallpox and yellow fever. The IHR, as they were subsequently renamed in 1969, required countries to alert WHO to any outbreak of these six diseases.

The IHR manifestly failed to protect global health security during the SARS outbreak of 2002–3. Their revision in 2005 represented a major step forward in international surveillance and security. The regulations now require countries to report any new illness or medical condition that presents (or could present) significant harm to human populations. It is the responsibility of countries to detect, assess and report events that could constitute a PHEIC.

The revised IHR of 2005 expanded the powers of WHO. The agency now had the responsibility to coordinate global surveillance efforts. It and it alone had the power to determine whether a PHEIC existed. And WHO could now advise countries about how best to respond to health emergencies as well as to mobilise financial resources to assist them in doing so. The IHR signalled the pre-eminence of global health over economics, of global governance over national sovereignty.

The IHR also invoked obligations on countries. WHO's member states now had to develop 'core capacities' to deal with major health emergencies. These capacities involved expanded laboratory networks, a trained health workforce, surveillance systems, response mechanisms, health service preparedness, risk communication, coordination procedures, and legislation and policy making – in other words, countries had the responsibility to ensure they had the full ability to detect, assess, report and respond to any new health hazard. The framework of global health security expressed in the IHR was crucial to WHO's pivotal role in calling out COVID-19 as an international health emergency.

But the idea of greater surveillance in society conjures up notions of threats to our privacy and liberty and even, as former UK Supreme Court justice Lord Sumption put it, a 'hysterical slide into a police state'.

Does greater surveillance truly imperil our freedom? In April, the *Financial Times* asked whether the advent of coronavirus apps meant that society was slipping gradually into a surveillance state. Apple and Google were working together to construct a wireless-based contact tracing system to inform someone if they crossed paths with a person who had had COVID-19. Aggressive detection of new cases, contact tracing and quarantine is the public health bulwark necessary to prevent subsequent waves of SARS-CoV-2 infection. Digital surveillance, the *FT* suggested, may become the greatest incursion into privacy our societies have ever seen.

But, so far at least, people seem sanguine. Governments have been surprised by the compliance of their usually dissenting and awkward publics. They – we – have willingly adhered to government demands to stay home under lockdown. Perhaps we will be equally docile when it comes to oversight of our daily lives.

Apple and Google promise that their electronic surveillance will be voluntary and anonymous. But if surveillance includes

cameras on every street corner, monitoring of credit card trans-
actions, tracking cell phone use, and having to scan QR health
codes before entering offices, public buildings and entertainment venues, one might not be surprised if the public becomes
sceptical about assurances that their privacy will be guaranteed.
And if information about your COVID-19 status is necessary
for digital surveillance to work, we will come perilously close
to introducing 'immunity passports'. An immunity passport
sounds a perfectly rational answer to the problem of a pandemic. Such a passport would allow you to go about your usual
life while others can be certain of their and your safety.

But immunity passports will also stigmatise those who are not
immune, creating a divided society and a class of non-immune
individuals who may be seen as a danger to public health.
Immunity passports will incentivise efforts to contract infection, with the attendant risk of severe, even fatal, illness. Far
better, surely, to accelerate work to produce a vaccine and offer
vaccination certificates instead. A vaccination certificate would
shift incentives away from infection and towards immunisation.

Enhanced surveillance for emerging infectious agents is
essential if future pandemics are to be prevented. Yet there are
reasons at least to understand the gravity of the social trend we
are likely to see in coming years. Michel Foucault, in his 1975
book *Discipline and Punish*, drew on Jeremy Bentham's idea
of the panopticon to identify a growing drift towards what he
called a 'disciplinary society'.

In its original conception, the panopticon was an architec-
tural design for a new type of prison.[3] Circular in nature, the

building would contain prison cells on its outer curve, while at the centre there would be the prison inspector's lodge. The inspector would be omnipresent, seen without being seen, while prisoners would (and should) always feel themselves under inspection. Bentham saw his panopticon – 'a new mode of obtaining power of mind over mind' – as being applicable to workhouses, poor-houses, factories, 'mad-houses', hospitals, schools and lazarettos (places of quarantine for those with the plague).

Bentham was the first utilitarian. He believed that humankind was governed by pain and pleasure. Utility was that property that tended 'to produce benefit, advantage, pleasure, good, or happiness … or … to prevent the happening of mischief, pain, evil, or unhappiness to the party whose interest is considered.' The panopticon was an expression of how to weave utilitarianism more deeply into the fabric of society. Total surveillance of the total population is the panopticon taken to its logical extreme. It is the ultimate expression of the disciplinary society. Coronavirus apps might be accelerating us towards Bentham's dream and Foucault's nightmare.

The IHR form a crucial instrument of this modern-day panopticon. They promulgate the idea and practice of omnipresent inspection. They embody a calculus of government oversight that insists on observation with minimal intrusion. They justify permanent surveillance in the name of pleasure over pain. The IHR seem like a clear example of a public good.

But is the apparatus of surveillance also indicative of something more sinister?

Foucault extended his interest in (and concern about) the disciplinary society by introducing the notion of 'biopolitics' – the politics of life. He meant 'the problems posed to governmental practice by phenomena characteristic of a set of living beings forming a population: health, hygiene, birthrate, life expectancy, race ... We know the increasing importance of these problems since the nineteenth century, and the political and economic issues they have raised up to the present'.[4]

The practical question was: how does a government regulate, manage and control its people? The answer? 'State control of the biological' and 'the emergence of techniques of power that were essentially centred on the body, on the individual body.' Foucault wrote that 'Biopolitics deals with the population, with the population as a political problem, as a problem that is at once scientific and political, as a biological problem and as power's problem.'[5] And the answer to this 'problem' of the population was 'bioregulation by the State'.

How do we reconcile the need for greater surveillance to diminish risks of future pandemics – the biopolitical disciplinary society – with a demand to protect the freedoms we have so come to take for granted? Does greater surveillance stand in opposition to our right to privacy? Is a disciplinary society, where government increasingly seeks ways to regulate public behaviour, inevitable in an Age of Pandemics? 'We'll keep your love affair secret, say contact tracers', ran one newspaper headline on the same day that one of the leading UK modelling scientists, Professor Neil Ferguson, resigned from SAGE for violating lockdown rules with his married lover.

Somehow we have to find an accommodation – an accommodation between liberty and scrutiny that is the most important public policy question facing Western society today.

There are no simple answers. COVID-19 has seen a rebirth of the state. Societies will see the state assume an ever greater role, from reconstructing state-sector economies to expanding social protection, from creating resilient health systems to transforming digital communication, from saving charities to investing even more generously in science. And as the state expands its reach, at the public's demand, so individual rights risk being curbed in the name of our common human security. We will be transformed into biopolitical citizens.

I don't fear greater state intrusion into our lives – the panopticonisation of society – provided that we insist that this intrusion is guided by some agreed principles, standards and values. There must be a commitment by government, first, to *universality and inalienability* – privacy protections must be afforded to everyone, without exception. Second, to *indivisibility* – our rights are interdependent: it is not for the state to determine which rights it will and will not guarantee. Third, to *equality and non-discrimination* – all human beings are equal in their dignity. And, fourth, and in some ways most importantly, to *transparency* – governments must be open about information and their decision-making. Many of the failures in COVID-19 responses had their origin in failures of transparency.

Must we accept and embrace the inevitability of a strengthened surveillance state and disciplinary society after COVID-19? I do not believe so. Instead, we should be committed to the creation of a vigilant state and society, one in which government and the public work together to identify, monitor and respond to new and emerging risks, while ensuring protections for our most cherished political and social rights.

Eternal vigilance truly is the price of freedom. We cannot afford to repeat the cycle of crisis, harm, action, complacency, neglect and subsequent vulnerability that followed SARS in 2002–3.

*

There is one troubling truth to this discussion of a dawning vigilant state and society. Uncertainty is its foundation.

One surprise as the COVID-19 epidemic unfolded was the immense uncertainty that surrounded what seemed like straightforward questions. Where did this new virus come from (there is early evidence that it was circulating before the outbreak in Wuhan)? Why were men more susceptible than women? Why were black and minority ethnic communities at special risk? Why were those living in care homes so vulnerable? What was a safe distance to maintain between individuals in the street, on public transport or in a queue outside a supermarket? Would wearing a face mask prevent infection or should the wearing of a mask be seen simply as an altruistic act, reducing the risk of someone who might be infected passing the virus on to someone else? Should schools be closed or, since children seemed to be least at risk of severe forms of COVID-19, could they remain open? Should governments shut their borders to prevent the introduction of the virus from other countries or was its importation so small as to constitute a negligible further risk when there was already ongoing community transmission of infection? After infection, what is the state of an individual's immunity and how long will that immunity last? Was having a BCG vaccination protective against developing COVID-19? Was hydroxychloroquine, a drug widely used to treat malaria, an effective medicine to treat SARS-CoV-2? And were lockdowns even necessary? Could a pandemic be managed by careful and consistent application of assiduous personal hygiene, physical distancing, and intensive testing, contact tracing and isolation?

These questions were asked, but precise and definitive answers were not immediately available. Instead, advice was given either in the absence of evidence or with only incomplete evidence on which to draw. More questions will inevitably follow. In some children, infection seems to cause a delayed-onset illness – Paediatric Inflammatory Multisystem Syndrome Temporally associated with SARS-CoV-2 (PIMS-TS) – that resembles a rare condition called Kawasaki disease. Why? And what will be the long-term outcomes? Those who are obese seem to be at greater risk of more severe disease. Again, why? And what can be done to protect those who are overweight?

It proved difficult for clinicians and politicians to manage risk in the face of such uncertainties. And these uncertainties only added to the difficulty of planning an exit from lockdown. Although answers will slowly emerge through further research, the (bio)political management of populations in peace, in conflict or at times of crisis will always be predicated on uncertainty. All the more reason, therefore, to have robust protections underpinning government actions in the vigilant state.

*

Two final reflections. Lockdowns around the world have increased some risks while reducing others. The dangers of domestic violence and child maltreatment were severely increased. The United Nations Population Fund estimated at least 15 million more cases of domestic violence as a result of pandemic restrictions. The fund's executive director, Natalia Kanem, called the impact of lockdowns on women 'totally calamitous'. And, in the UK, calls raising concerns about child abuse rose by 20 per cent.

Disruption of health systems and services in low- and middle-income countries is expected to be especially devastating. Timothy Roberton and his colleagues from the Johns Hopkins Bloomberg School of Public Health calculated that the pandemic lockdowns would lead, at the very least, to 253,000 additional deaths of children under five and 12,200 additional maternal deaths across 118 of the poorest countries in the world.[6] The worst case scenario they studied is almost incomprehensible in its tragic proportions – a further 1.2 million child deaths and 56,700 maternal deaths.

The wider economic and human costs of lockdowns have been plain for all to see. In the UK, the Bank of England predicted the deepest recession for 300 years, together with a sharp rise in unemployment and with no prospect of a quick recovery. Economies cannot be put on hold for long.

Yet, paradoxically, there have also been unexpected benefits. The incidence of road traffic injuries fell. Air quality improved. Greenhouse gas emissions declined. Some estimates put the numbers of deaths averted from these risk reductions in the tens of thousands.

How does a society, even a vigilant society, now navigate between these losses and gains? How do we retain, as far as we can, the benefits we have accrued while eliminating the disadvantages?

Slavoj Žižek, in perhaps the first serious response to COVID-19's implications, predicts the possibility of an 'alternate society' emerging.[7] Although Žižek doesn't believe the pandemic will make us any wiser, he is surely right to argue that 'even horrible events can have unpredictable positive consequences.' He suggests that the responses of governments have made us all communists now. He doesn't mean communist in the Soviet sense. He means communist as an expression of 'new forms of local and global solidarity', 'abandoning market mechanisms' to solve social problems, and avoiding a 'new barbarism'. But his conclusion that COVID-19 has precipitated the 'disintegration of trust' in governments, exposing 'their basic impotence', hardly heralds the moment for a rebirth of humanity.

Ulrich Beck's answer to the dilemmas posed by a risk society was to encourage a more vigorous culture of self-criticism:

Only when medicine opposes medicine, nuclear physics opposes nuclear physics, human genetics opposes human genetics, or information technology opposes information technology can the future that is being brewed up in the test-tube become intelligible and evaluable for the outside world. Enabling self-criticism in all its forms is not some sort of danger, but probably the *only way* that the mistakes that would sooner or later destroy our world can be detected in advance.[8]

The seismologist Lucy Jones put it this way in her book *The Big Ones*: 'Science works only when its practitioners are free to argue opposite sides.' We need to foster better and more informed conversations (and criticisms) about our present and future, about the kinds of people we want to be, about the kind of society we wish to inhabit, and about what we owe to one another.

There is often resistance to this call for greater self-criticism. At the height of the pandemic in the UK, when unfavourable comparisons were being drawn between Britain's response to COVID-19 and that of other European countries, Professor Chris Whitty, England's chief medical officer, argued that

We must learn lessons at the right point. But what you don't do, frankly, is do that in the middle of something. We are nowhere near the end of this epidemic. We are through the first phase of this, but there is a very long way to run for every country in the world on this. And I think let's not go charging in on who's won and who's lost at this point ... Let's do the post-action review, which we absolutely must, at the right moment and we are definitely not at that stage yet.

Now is not the right time to review what went right and what went wrong. That was a common refrain from government scientists and politicians as the pandemic unfolded.

Indeed, those of my colleagues within the medical community who did raise their voices to comment on (and, indeed, to criticise) the UK government's response were frequently 'hammered' by more senior colleagues who urged silence, fearing perhaps retribution in the form of lost government research grant income or future exclusion from powerful and prestigious leadership roles and committees. But those who criticised didn't want 'scalps'; they didn't want to apportion blame to individuals. Instead, they wanted to hold government accountable for its decisions. As one professor of global health, who had spoken out but had been pressured by their own institution to stay silent, wrote to me, 'I just don't understand why academics can't speak freely. Freedom of speech? So many senior people sitting quiet. While thousands die.'

Perhaps we need a different attitude of mind. It is common today to praise the optimist and condemn the pessimist. Who wants to listen to those who spread nothing but gloom? Surely it is better to be a boosterist – to view the world more positively, adopt a can-do approach, be enthusiastic and fearless, believe that our common problems will be solved. We can discover new drugs to disable a virus. We can devise a new vaccine to protect against future infection. We can eliminate the threat of a further pandemic. Maybe.

Yet optimism can also blind us, imbue us with a sense of power and overconfidence, and mask real dangers that need to be embraced, understood, and addressed with humility and care. Human beings are condemned to suffer from optimism bias. We tend to overestimate the likelihood that good things will happen in life.

Benjamin Fondane (1898–1944) was a Romanian Jew who emigrated to France in 1923. He was deported to Auschwitz in 1944 and killed just two weeks before the Soviets arrived the following year to liberate the camp. In his fragmentary writings, Fondane questioned the influence of excessive rationalism as a solution to the predicaments facing humankind:

> If the final result of four centuries of humanism and the apotheosis of science has been only a return of the worst horrors … the fault lies perhaps with humanism itself, which was too lacking in pessimism, which staked too much on the separate and divine intellect, and neglected more than it ought to have the real man, whom we had treated as an angel only to finally reduce him to a level lower than the beasts.[9]

An appeal for greater pessimism in our dealings with the world may not feel like an inspiring call to arms to avert the next pandemic. But if the scientists and politicians who gave advice and took decisions on our behalf had adopted a little more pessimism in their predictions and policies, the deaths of hundreds of thousands of their fellow citizens around the world would have been avoided.

Pessimism need not kill our hopes for a better future. Hope is a feeling of desire for a particular outcome in our lives. We can protect and, indeed, intensify our hopes through a perspective that does not mask the worst that can happen to us.

*

As we turn to the future, there will be a temptation to say we should be grateful for what we once had before COVID-19. We will be encouraged to be appreciative of the orderliness of our past existence, to be thankful for the harmony of our disharmonies. The status quo ante will be exalted, even glorified. We must not be tolerant of past conventions. There is a place between normality and utopia, a place towards which it is worth striving. It is up to us now to discover that place. As Herbert Marcuse observed, tolerance 'protects the already established machinery of discrimination'; it is 'an instrument for the continuation of servitude'. If the hope after COVID-19 is for a more humane society – a worthy hope given the devastation this virus has wreaked – we must work hard to cultivate our sensibility for intolerance.

# 7

# Towards the Next Pandemic

The time has come when nations must either accept a hideous death or else care for their bodies as they care for their minds, when governments must embrace the material as well as the rational development of the human race and concern themselves as much with the clothing, diet, gymnastics, and indeed the flesh of the governed, in all its forms, as they do, or are supposed to do, with the people's intelligence.

Michel Chevalier (1832), quoted by François Delaporte,
*Disease and Civilization* (1986)

COVID-19 brought a divided world together and then divided it still further. The international community failed to unite to defeat the worst consequences of this pandemic. As UN Secretary General António Guterres noted, COVID-19 unleashed a 'tsunami of hate and xenophobia, scapegoating and scaremongering'. We are now living through a period of unparalleled political, economic, and social anxiety and instability.

The virus that caused COVID-19 isn't going away. It will be with us for a very long time to come. The best we can hope for is peaceful coexistence. There will likely be public inquiries in every country badly scarred by the deaths of so many thousands of citizens. There will certainly be global investigations into the origin, course and outcome of this pandemic. Long lists of recommendations will be made. Some may even be acted upon. The COVID-19 crisis of 2020 will give rise to a renewed sense of the centrality of health for modern society.

That said, Slavoj Žižek is right: disasters can be catalysts for significant and surprising social and political change. Here is what societies must do if they are to prevent the most extreme depredations of the next pandemic.

Within countries, the regime of science policymaking will be questioned and overhauled – devising mechanisms to assemble a wider array of specialists to assess and judge risks transparently and more self-critically. Not only will the afferent input to government be improved, but also the efferent response will be optimised to be faster and more decisive. Resilient health systems will be constructed to be better prepared to withstand the shocks of sudden new diseases. Health and social care will be unified into a single healthcare system. A redistribution of esteem will recognise (and reward) key workers. Inequality will rise on the public's list of political priorities. In 2013, the UK's prime minister, Boris Johnson (then mayor of London), argued that 'inequality was essential' for society's success. 'The spirit of envy', he said, was a 'valuable spur to economic activity'. That view will no longer be acceptable. Governments will attack inequality with every fibre of their political being. And countries with live-animal markets will begin to close them down.

Internationally, countries, initially without the support of the US, will work together to strengthen and reform WHO, the only international agency that can lead and coordinate the global response to a pandemic. To enhance vigilance for new infectious threats, countries will come to view health not merely as a domestic concern but as a foreign policy issue foundational to national security. They will collaborate to ensure that all nations make progress towards the goal of universal health coverage, since individual health security is indispensable for global health security. Countries will cooperate to share data and defeat disinformation. And they will find ways, slowly, to strengthen their accountability to meet the stringent requirements of the IHR.

But beyond these important and specific technical advances to enhance human security – advances that will deliver immeasurable co-benefits to society – there will also be momentous changes to the trajectory of humankind. Arundhati Roy has described COVID-19 as 'a portal, a gateway between one world and the next'.[1] What might that other world look like?

*COVID-19 will change societies.* COVID-19 has revealed the mortal weaknesses of our nations. The economic costs – collapsed businesses, rising unemployment, declining growth – will threaten the future of an entire generation for decades to come. The vigilant state and society will become the new normal. We must embrace it. The threat this pandemic posed will emphasise the importance of protecting and strengthening the health of civilisations as well as communities – what one might call our planetary health. Our museums are filled with the relics of ancient peoples who once thought their societies were stable and robust. The fragility of our civilisations has been brought into stark relief by COVID-19. The political, economic, social, technological and environmental determinants of a stable and sustainable society will become matters of the utmost political importance. The idea of progress will be redefined – reversal is a permanent possibility. The chief economist of the Bank of England has argued that societies have underestimated the importance of social capital as a counter-cyclical stabilizer.[2] Policymakers will pay more attention to strengthening social capital.

*COVID-19 will change governments.* Politicians have understood that a pandemic is a political crisis and not merely a health crisis – pandemics demand leadership at the highest political level. Presidents and prime ministers have also felt, sometimes through their own illnesses, the responsibility they have to protect the lives and livelihoods of their peoples: relying on markets to solve society's problems is not enough. A country's political parties and civil service will recruit more scientists to their ranks. Science literacy will be a necessary requirement for governing. Governments will have to find better means for leadership and coordination, regionally and globally. They will understand the importance of public trust for public order. The US government will eventually be reintegrated into a new system of global collaboration, but not with Donald Trump as president.

*COVID-19 will change publics.* Citizens will demand stronger health services and public health systems. Our expectations will rise. We will welcome the rebirth of the state. Health may become an obsession as well as a fear. Concerns about our health and about the risk of further pandemics will trigger debates about the organisation of society. Publics will no longer view disease as a pathology of the body. We will see disease as a pathology of society. People will demand stronger systems of social protection, especially for the most vulnerable. We will rediscover the idea of community. And we will come to accept the risk of infection – and death – as a necessary trade-off to win back our liberties.

*COVID-19 will change medicine.* The concept of One Health will become a new priority. One Health recognises that the health of humans and the health of animals are intricately connected. Health workers and their institutions will have a larger voice in society. More health workers will be recruited and educated. Public health systems will be strengthened. The well-being of health workers will be taken more seriously. They will sharpen their demands of politicians and ask for greater input into political decision-making. More attention will be paid to the health of key populations – older people living in care homes, black and minority ethnic communities, migrants and refugees, and those living in circumstances of pervasive deprivation. The way in which care is delivered will be transformed by digital technology, especially in primary care. Investments in medical (and especially in public health) science will be enhanced.

*COVID-19 will change science.* Research will speed up, and it will be fully integrated into clinical care. COVID-19 proved that science – and clinical trials in particular – can be done in the middle of a pandemic storm. Research will usher in a new range of drugs and vaccines to treat and prevent COVID-19.

Remdesivir has already received emergency approval by the US Food and Drug Administration. Further antivirals are being studied. And vaccines have entered early clinical trials. The dangers of therapeutic and vaccine nationalism will be severe. Means will be found to ensure fair access to new health technologies. A guiding ethical principle in the science of COVID-19 will be equity – world populations must have equal opportunity to benefit from the products of scientific research. Evidence will assume far greater importance in political decision-making. Transparency of that evidence must become the norm rather than the exception. New fields of knowledge will be created.

Each of us will have our own observations and interpretations about COVID-19 too.

I worry that our generation of political leaders will be unable to grasp the opportunity presented to it. There is little sign that any leader is currently willing to transcend their sovereign interests. On the contrary, there is ample evidence of an emerging and more ruthless inward-looking nationalism. If that is the path our world takes, there is no prospect for preventing the worst excesses of a future pandemic.

I worry that many of the issues shaping our future, which were discussed before COVID-19 struck, will be pushed to one side – poverty, malnutrition, lack of access to education, gender inequality (and inequalities more broadly), the climate emergency, polluted oceans, and war and conflict. You might recognise this list of concerns. They make up some of the Sustainable Development Goals (SDGs), an extraordinary set of political commitments supported by all nations, with a deadline to deliver by 2030. The SDGs are a promise we are making to our children. COVID-19 must not divert us – or not divert us too much – from fulfilling the objective of sustainable human development. We must not pass on the costs of COVID-19 to the next generation.

I worry that one result of COVID-19 will be not only greater US detachment from world affairs (the world needs a strongly engaged US government if we are to succeed in meeting the SDGs) but also a repudiation of China. The overt racism that COVID-19 brought down on China is a mistake as well as a misfortune. China can make an important contribution to solving some of the deepest problems we face as a human community. China's scientific acumen, its ability to innovate, and a desire among its best minds to collaborate – all distinct qualities that I have witnessed grow in Chinese medicine and medical science over two decades – should be welcomed and harnessed for the common good. Binding China closer to the international community will promote the emergence of common norms among nations. This convergence in values and behaviour was one result of the successful control of SARS in 2002–3. It would be an immense missed opportunity if the mishandling of COVID-19 led to a new phase of dissolution among nations.

I worry that we will lose our capacity to be shocked. Albert Camus, in his 1947 appeal to doctors fighting the plague, wrote, 'You must not, you must never, get used to seeing people die like flies in our streets, the way they are now, and the way they have always done ever since the plague received its name in Athens.'[3] We must retain our capacity to be horrified by the incompetence of governments, the corruption of entrusted power and the collusion of elites. And we must be prepared to act on those feelings of horror.

I worry that fear will become a new organising principle of society. That physical distance will evolve as a norm in our relationships. That trust between us will disintegrate. Seats on buses and trains will distance us. Cinemas and theatres will contract their audiences and perhaps their power to move us. Bars and restaurants will demand segregation over association. Lars Svendsen argues that 'Fear has become a basic characteristic of our entire culture.'4 What if we create a society that prefers to diminish evil instead of encouraging good? Svendsen points out that fear is closely linked to uncertainty. But, as I have sought to show, uncertainty is foundational to our future. If we allow the fear of uncertainty to engulf us, the costs to life may create an unacceptable deficit for living.

And I worry that we will forget – forget the facts and lessons of COVID-19, just as we forgot the facts and lessons of SARS in 2002–3. Over 300,000 deaths worldwide surely counts as a significant event in the human story. We should at least consider whether we have an obligation to remember. Of course, families will recall the individual lives lost. But I am asking something more. Do we as a global community have an obligation to remember – not only as an aggregate of individual memories but also as a shared memory? I believe we do, partly because this shared memory is what we owe to those who died and partly because we need to remind ourselves what we must do to prevent this avoidable tragedy from repeating itself. Whether through physical memorials, commemorative ceremonies or communal institutions, the construction of this shared memory matters, since, as Avishai Margalit points out, 'a proper community of memory may help shape a nation.'[5]

COVID-19 has provided us with an opportunity to rethink the ethical basis of our society. The virus took so many lives. We can't allow ourselves to return to our old worlds as if that fact can somehow be elided. To honour the lives lost we have to live differently. What we face now is not only a political predicament of enormous proportions. We also face a moral provocation.

Capitalism has many virtues. But the intense version of capitalism that has emerged over the past forty years has weakened something essential in the social fabric of our societies. Those weaknesses contributed to the tragic toll of deaths. After COVID-19, it is no longer acceptable to see people as means rather than ends. Once we have resuscitated ourselves after this pandemic, can we seize a moment to redefine our values and our goals together? For we did seem to learn to value one another more during this pandemic. Although isolated, we edged closer together. We took time to ask about each other's health. We relaxed our expectations and became more generous in our praise. We explicitly gave priority to our wellbeing over our wealth.

\*

There is no single final all-encompassing lesson to learn from the COVID-19 pandemic. There is no ultimate meaning to be found in the lives needlessly lost – except for this thought perhaps.

COVID-19 is not an event. Instead, it has defined the beginning of a new epoch. It took a virus to connect us in life and in death. We understand now, I think, our extraordinary interdependence and unity as a species. Yet our world is organised and ordered by separation, by partition – countries and continents, languages and faiths, political systems and ideological allegiances.

We surely have to use this occasion to resist and to challenge the past mood for estrangement and prejudice. We have to use this time for solidarity, for mutual respect and mutual concern. My health depends on your health. Your health depends on my health. We cannot escape one another. The liberties that we prize so highly depend on the health of all of us. We cannot say that the politics and priorities of my country are of no concern to you. They are, and legitimately so. Just as the politics and priorities of your country are a legitimate interest of mine. Sovereignty is dead.

The post-COVID-19 age will usher in a new era of social and political relations, one in which our liberties will be achieved through new means of cooperation and communication. One can be proud of one's national culture and identity. But COVID-19 also shows the importance we should attach to our global human identity. We are social beings. We are political beings. COVID-19 has taught us that we are mutual beings too.

# Notes

## Chapter 1  From Wuhan to the World

1 Jasper Fuk-Woo Chan et al., A familial cluster of pneumonia associated with the 2019 novel coronavirus indicating person-to-person transmission, *The Lancet*, 24 January 2020.

2 Chaolin Huang et al., Clinical features of patients infected with 2019 novel coronavirus in Wuhan, China, *The Lancet*, 24 January 2020.

3 Joseph T. Wu et al., Nowcasting and forecasting the potential domestic and international spread of the 2019-nCoV outbreak originating in Wuhan, China, *The Lancet*, 31 January 2020.

4 Adam Kucharski, *The Rules of Contagion: Why Things Spread – and Why They Stop* (London: Profile Books, 2020).

5 Adam J. Kucharski et al., Early dynamics of transmission and control of COVID-19, *Lancet Infectious Diseases*, 11 March 2020.

6 Novel Coronavirus Pneumonia Emergency Response Epidemiology Team, The epidemiological characteristics of an outbreak of 2019 novel coronavirus diseases (COVID-19) – China 2020, *China CDC Weekly*, 2/8 (2020): 113–22.

7 Kiesha Prem et al., The effect of control strategies to reduce social mixing on outcomes of COVID-19 epidemic in Wuhan, China, *Lancet Public Health*, 25 March 2020.

8 Benjamin J. Cowling et al., Impact assessment of non-pharmaceutical interventions against coronavirus disease 2019 and influenza in Hong Kong, *The Lancet*, 17 April 2020.

9 Samantha Brooks et al., The psychological impact of quarantine and how to reduce it, *The Lancet*, 26 February 2020.

## Chapter 2  Why Were We Not Prepared?

1 Ian Boyd, We practised for a pandemic, but didn't brace, *Nature*, 30 March 2020, p. 9.

2 Institute of Medicine, *Learning from SARS: Preparing for the Next Disease Outbreak* (Washington, DC: National Academies Press, 2004).

3 Ibid., p. 37.

4 David P. Fidler, *SARS, Governance and the Globalization of Disease* (Basingstoke: Palgrave Macmillan, 2004).

5 Nirmal Kandel et al., Health security capacities in the context of COVID-2019 outbreak, *The Lancet*, 18 March 2020.

## Chapter 3  Science: The Paradox of Success and Failure

1 Chaolin Huang et al., Clinical features of patients infected with 2019 novel coronavirus in Wuhan, China, *The Lancet*, 24 January 2020.

2 Jasper Fuk-Woo Chan et al., A familial cluster of pneumonia

associated with the 2019 novel coronavirus indicating person-to-person transmission, *The Lancet*, 24 January 2020.

3  Roujian Lu et al., Genomic characterisation and epidemiology of 2019 novel coronavirus: implications for virus origins and receptor binding, *The Lancet*, 29 January 2020.

4  Joseph T. Wu et al., Nowcasting and forecasting the potential domestic and international spread of the 2019-nCoV outbreak originating in Wuhan, China, *The Lancet*, 31 January 2020.

5  Huijun Chen et al., Clinical characteristics and intrauterine vertical transmission potential of COVID-19 infection in nine pregnant women, *The Lancet*, 12 February 2020.

6  Nanshan Chen et al., Epidemiological and clinical characteristics of 99 cases of 2019 novel coronavirus pneumonia in Wuhan, China, *The Lancet*, 29 January 2020.

7  Xiaobo Yang et al., Clinical course and outcomes of critically ill patients with SARS-CoV-2 pneumonia in Wuhan, China, *Lancet Respiratory Medicine*, 21 February 2020.

8  WHO, *Report of the WHO–China Joint Mission on Coronavirus Disease 2019 (COVID-19), 16–24 February 2020*, www.who.int/docs/default-source/coronaviruse/who-china-joint-mission-on-covid-19-final-report.pdf.

9  Anup Bastola et al., The first 2019 novel coronavirus case in Nepal, *Lancet Infectious Diseases*, 10 February 2020.

10  William Silverstein et al., First imported case of 2019 novel coronavirus in Canada, presenting as mild pneumonia, *The Lancet*, 13 February 2020.

11  Andrea Remuzzi and Giuseppe Remuzzi, COVID-19 and Italy: what next? *The Lancet*, 12 March 2020.

12  Isaac Ghinai et al., First known person-to-person transmission of severe acute respiratory syndrome coronavirus 2 (SARS-CoV-2) in the USA, *The Lancet*, 12 March 2020.

13  Rachael Pung et al., Investigation of three clusters of COVID-19 in Singapore, *The Lancet*, 16 March 2020.

14  Remuzzi and Remuzzi, COVID-19 and Italy: what next?

15  Laurie Garrett, *The Coming Plague: Newly Emerging Diseases in a World out of Balance* (Harmondsworth: Penguin, 1994).

16  Institute of Medicine, *Learning from SARS: Preparing for the Next Disease Outbreak* (Washington, DC: National Academies Press, 2004).

17  Lucy Jones, *The Big Ones: How Natural Disasters Have Shaped Us (and What We can Do about Them)* (London: Icon Books, 2018).

18  Independent Scientific Advisory Group for Emergencies, *COVID-19: What Are the Options for the UK? Recommendations for Government based on an Open and Transparent Examination of the Scientific Evidence*, 12 May 2020, www.independentsage. org/wp-content/uploads/2020/05/The-Independent-SAGE-Report.pdf.

## Chapter 4  First Lines of Defence

1  Simiao Chen et al., Fangcang shelter hospitals: a novel concept for responding to public health emergencies, *The Lancet*, 2 April 2020.

2  Amitava Banerjee et al., Estimating excess 1-year mortality associated with the COVID-19 pandemic according to underlying conditions and age, *The Lancet*, 12 May 2020.

## Chapter 5   The Politics of COVID-19

1   Jacques Ellul, *Propaganda: The Formation of Men's Attitudes* (New York: Alfred A. Knopf, 1965).

2   Didier Fassin, *Life: A Critical User's Manual* (Cambridge: Polity, 2018).

## Chapter 6   The Risk Society Revisited

1   Ulrich Beck, *Risk Society: Towards a New Modernity*, trans. Mark Ritter (London: Sage, [1986] 1992), p. 183.

2   Ibid., p. 59.

3   Jeremy Bentham, *The Panopticon Writings* (London: Verso, 1995).

4   Michel Foucault, *The Birth of Biopolitics: Lectures at the Collège de France, 1978–79* (Basingstoke: Palgrave Macmillan, 2008).

5   Michel Foucault, *Society Must Be Defended: Lectures at the Collège de France, 1975–76* (London: Penguin, 2004).

6   Timothy Roberton et al., Early estimates of the indirect effects of the COVID-19 pandemic on maternal and child mortality in low-income and middle-income countries, *Lancet Global Health*, 12 May 2020.

7   Slavoj Žižek, *Pandemic! COVID-19 Shakes the World* (Cambridge: Polity, 2020).

8   Beck, *Risk Society*, p. 234.

9   Benjamin Fondane, *Existential Monday* (New York: New York Review of Books, 2016).

## Chapter 7  Towards the Next Pandemic

1 Arundhati Roy, The pandemic is a portal, *Financial Times*, 3 April 2020.

2 Andy Haldane, Reweaving the social fabric after the crisis, *Financial Times*, 24 April 2020.

3 Albert Camus, How to survive a plague, *Sunday Times*, 10 May 2020.

4 Lars Svendsen, *A Philosophy of Fear*, trans. John Irons (London: Reaktion Books, 2008).

5 Avishai Margalit, *The Ethics of Memory* (Cambridge, MA: Harvard University Press, 2002).